Other book

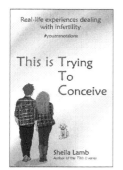

Infertility sucks doesn't it? You shouldn't feel alone whilst on your journey to having a baby. Read real-life experiences and thoughts from the fabulous TTC community, who want to support you and let you know that #youarenotalone. Available in print and as an ebook.

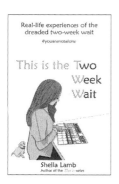

Are you about to go through the dreaded two-week wait? Whether this is your first or you've been here before, this wait has to be one of the hardest times on the journey to becoming a parent.
Available in print and as an ebook.

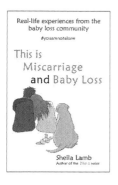

If you've experienced a miscarriage or baby loss, I'm so sorry. Nothing can take your pain away, but we hope that our words of emotional support and empathy help you to know that you are not alone.
Available in print and as an ebook.

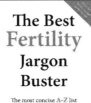

The Best Fertility Jargon Buster

The most concise A–Z list of fertility abbreviations and acronyms you will ever need.

SHEILA LAMB

Feeling overwhelmed by the infertility language? Confused with what the abbreviations and acronyms stand for on social media, Facebook groups and websites? All is made clear in this invaluable resource. Available as a FREE ebook – download from www.mfsbooks.co.uk

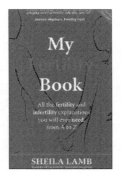

My [...] Book

All the fertility and infertility explanations you will ever need from A to Z

SHEILA LAMB

Are you stressed navigating the world of conception? Do you feel overwhelmed by the sheer amount of infertility information available online? This comprehensive, jargon-free book explains over 200 medical and non-medical terms. Available in print and as an ebook.

Real-life experiences of going through fertility treatments

#youarenotalone

This is IVF and other Fertility Treatments

Sheila Lamb

Author of the *This is* series

Published in 2020 by MFSBooks.com

Print ISBN 978-1-9993035-4-9

A CIP catalogue record for this book is available from the British Library.

Dedicated to every woman and man who has been through fertility treatment to start or grow their family

Disclaimer

This book is intended purely to share people's real-life experiences of fertility treatments, such as IVF, IUI, ICSI and ovulation stimulation, offering words of support and comfort. It is written in their words; their experience is not medical advice. It does not replace the advice and information from your healthcare specialist, such as your doctor, nurse or other health expert. Nor is it a substitute for counselling or coaching. If brand names are mentioned, the author does not endorse the product or company.

The author does not accept liability for readers who choose to self-prescribe.

The information provided must not be used for diagnosing or treating a health problem or disease.

This information was correct at the time of publication and has been interpreted by the author.

Acknowledgements

This book, and the 'This is' series it is part of, would not exist if it wasn't for the women and men who are part of the most amazing and supportive community that ever existed. It wasn't until I joined Instagram after publishing: *My Fertility Book – All the Fertility and Infertility Explanations you will ever need, from A to Z*, that I realised what 'community' actually means. Although my rollercoaster journey of infertility treatment ended happily several years ago, it has helped me to accept the emotions that come with all areas of infertility, and are still part of me.

My thanks, firstly, go to my miracle, rainbow daughter Jessica, who means the world to me and is my reason for writing and helping the TTC and baby loss community. Secondly, each contributor saw my vision for this series and has kindly shared their emotions in order support you. I appreciate each and every one of them, especially as most of them I have never met IRL, only on Instagram or Facebook. So, in alphabetical order: Adriana Michael @stateofsantosha, Amelia @infertilebruises, Aysha O'Connor, Becky Kearns @ definingmum, Caren @themissinghare, Carla Heilbron @ Carlafertility.coach, Claire Ingle @ivfatwork, Dany Griffiths @freedomfertilityformula, Devon Baeza @the_fertility_ finance_coach, Eloise @fertility_help_hub, Emma Manser @ finding_my_rainbow_, Erin Bulcao @mybeautifulblunder, @ fertilit-arty, Gareth James, Jessica Hepburn @jessica_hepburn_, Clare Deakin @iwannabemamabear, Jo Sinclair @jo.sinclair. resilience.reborn, Jocelyn @motheringsolo, Julianne Boutaleb @parenthoodinmind, Justine Bold @justinebold, Katy Jenkins @thejstartshere, Kelly @ivf.ninja, Lauren Juggler Crook, Leah Irby @leahirby, Lisa Penny @fertilityism, Lisa White @ivf.manifesting.a.miracle, Chiemi Rajamahendran @ missconceptioncoach, Monica Bivas @monicabivas, Monica Cox @findingfertility, @mrandmrsivf, Natalie Silverman @ fertilitypoddy, Rachael Casella @mylifeof_love, Rachel Cathan @rachelcathancounselling, Sandi Friedlos @SandiFriedlos, Sophie Martin @the.infertile.midwife, Suzanne Minnis

@thebabygaim and @the.swim.team, If you want to connect with any of these lovely people, go to the 'Resources' section at the end of the book where you will find their contact information.

The book cover was illustrated by the author and illustrator, Sheila Alexander, who was so supportive and patient as I stumbled to explain what I wanted for this book and the series. We both very much hope you relate to the woman who is having an injection for the fertility treatment, whilst her concerned fur-baby looks on.

Sheila Alexander is the author of: IF: A Memoir of Infertility, a graphic novel about her infertility treatment using in-vitro fertilization (IVF). She lives in Massachusetts with her husband, son, dog, and parrot. She holds a master's degree in education and is a minor in fine art from Lesley University. By day, she works as a teacher, where she shares her love of comic books with her students. She believes that books have the power to change lives, so she published her first book, in the hope that it would help others who are going through infertility treatments. For more information visit her website: www.sheilaalexanderart.com or follow her on Instagram @sheilaalexanderart.

Sheila also captured parts of this journey in the illustrations you'll find inside the book, as did the author and illustrator Phillip Reed, who created the illustrations in the other books in the This is series and *My Fertility Book*. He can be contacted on philr@live.co.uk and Instagram @the_phillustrator.

I'd also like to thank the following people who have encouraged and supported me to put my This Is series of books together: my parents John and Freda, my sister Judy Marell, Paul Lamb, Michelle Starkey, Claudia Sievers, Angie Conlon, Maria Bagao, Carla McMahon, numerous fertility advocates and my author writing group.

Contents

Contents

Introduction

If you find yourself reading this book, you have my heartfelt support, because IVF (in vitro fertilisation) or any other fertility treatment is not what you'd expect to go through in order to have a baby. It's a shock and it's scary, I know, I've been there. Or, perhaps you're reading this because someone you care about has gifted it to you, or recommended it, so you can understand why fertility treatments are so stressful.

Unless you have an identified medical condition, such as blocked Fallopian tubes, you might have tried to get pregnant for many years, and now you're going through IVF, a variation of IVF or IUI (intrauterine insemination) in the hope there'll be positive results. Fortunately, it does work for many, not necessarily the first time they try it, but eventually. However, for others, fertility treatment doesn't result in them bringing home a baby.

With the first IUI or IVF cycle, you may well feel relief, because at last you're nearer to your goal and doing something constructive. You may also be worried that it won't work, and many aren't willing to put all their energy and money into something that's not guaranteed. But you're desperate and I understand that. You won't have got to this point without going through plenty of heartache – your period arriving without fail, piles of negative pregnancy tests, taunting pregnancy announcements from others, and quite possibly miscarriage. Now you're putting all your trust, dedication and quite likely your savings, into the science that might be how you get to take home your baby. You are not alone.

The advancements made in fertility treatments since the first IVF baby was born in the UK in 1978 has been incredible, and with more than eight million babies born following IVF, it's resulted in many grateful parents. What will always remain the same is that indescribable urge to have a child and the deep sadness we feel when it doesn't happen. That's the reason why we embark on IUI or IVF; why we inject ourselves with hormones, go through the indignity of scans of our reproductive system, sometimes needing painful surgery (women and men), have conversations with our partners we never dreamt we'd have, and pay out money that was meant for our children's wellbeing and future, not to create them.

Often before we embark on fertility treatment, we have to make choices and lifestyle changes. Your religion may be against IVF, so you need to process this first. Most clinics insist on a potential mother being below a certain weight and BMI (body mass index), so you may need diet and lifestyle changes – all the while knowing other overweight women conceive naturally. Becoming pregnant is personal and you may not have told anyone, so when it's months or years later, you may still not want to share the start of your IVF journey. Everyone's reasons are valid and vary from not wanting to worry their family, preferring not to explain why they can't get pregnant naturally, or not wanting to get theirs and other people's hopes up. Or you might tell others that you're now starting fertility treatment because you know they'll be supportive. We're all different and there's no right or wrong way.

Whether you're doing your first cycle or you're on your fifth, it's a nerve-wracking time, because so much is invested in each cycle. Fertility treatments take over your life; attending clinic appointments, blood tests, investigations and scans, then the endless waiting – for the results, to start your injections, for follicles to develop and your womb lining to thicken, to see how many eggs have fertilised, and finally for your embryos to develop as they should and for one to be put safely back where it belongs, in your womb. The final wait is roughly two weeks, commonly called the 'two-week wait' and abbreviated to TWW or 2WW – at the end, you either get a positive pregnancy test – possibly the first one ever – or you don't. And that's another story – illustrated in the book: *This is the Two Week Wait.*

Finding it challenging to have a baby is a life-changing experience for most. It certainly was for me. Even though we were eventually successful, this experience was very much part of my life and what has made me, me. Like a lot of people when this happens, I wanted to give something back to those who also find themselves on this path, to offer help and support. Coming from a medical background – I was a nurse and midwife many years ago – I appreciated that understanding the medical terms whilst going through such a stressful time is difficult, so I wrote my first book: *My Fertility Book: all the fertility and infertility explanations you will ever need, from A to Z* and published it in 2018. It's a jargon-free glossary of over two hundred medical and non-medical terms, with illustrations to help explain and cartoons to bring a smile to your face.

Most fertility terms have acronyms or are abbreviated, such as AMH, BBT, and 6DP5DT, and are often used on social media, forums, online groups and websites. So, I wrote a FREE eBook called: *The Best Fertility Jargon Buster: the most concise A-Z list of fertility abbreviations and acronyms you will ever need.* Download this FREE eBook here: www.mfsbooks.co.uk

Most people don't talk about their struggle to conceive and that they're going through fertility treatment, so many find support and comfort online from strangers who often become friends. Sharing feelings is comforting as you realise that you're not alone, and it's okay to feel worried, anxious, and negative one minute and then positive and optimistic the next. Women and men feel supported, boosted and, most important, understood and validated by a community of other people who also find themselves part of an intimate global group. Nobody wants to be in a group of 'failure to conceive' people, but when you find yourself part of it, boy, they have your back.

It was reading the posts in these communities that gave me the idea of collating all these lovely, warm, supportive, virtual hugging words into a book. Then, if you find during your cycle that it's all getting a bit too much, reach for this guide and read about those who've been there before you. They'll help get you through it.

Practically all the contributors have experienced fertility treatment, and if they haven't, they've worked with men and women who've been trying to conceive for years. They've kindly given up their time to share their own experiences. Each quoted extract is in the voice of the contributor.

Remember, there's no right or wrong way to deal with IUI and IVF, but these inspiring women and men hope that their words will in some way help you – until you hold your longed-for baby in your arms, and start your lives together as a family.

With Love

Sheila xx

Visit my website at www.mfsbooks.com

A letter to someone due to have IVF

Dear Friend

I'm so sorry you're reading this book because I know how much you want a baby and I understand that your journey till now won't have been easy. I know you're fed up of waiting to become a parent, and that every baby announcement on social media hurts more than the last one. It's been a long road to get to the point of having to undergo fertility treatment, such as IVF. (I'll generally only mention IVF because this is the commonest known fertility treatment, but the emotions felt are the same for all treatments).

If this is your first IVF cycle, you're probably experiencing a huge range of emotions – from excitement that at last you're doing something constructive to get pregnant, to feeling scared that your first cycle won't work. And this is all completely normal.

Our reasons for receiving IVF are varied and this makes it harder for people to understand what we go through. And because people don't fully understand what's involved, they can't possibly give us the support we dearly need. I bet you didn't know much about IVF before finding yourself thrust into the midst of it. I certainly didn't.

Most of the contributors in this book have undergone at least one IUI or IVF cycle. One contributor had eleven cycles and still never took a baby home. They've written from their hearts, sharing their thoughts and experiences because they understand how difficult it is to go through this process, and how much there is riding on it. They want you to know that you're not alone and we're all stronger together.

We understand how frustrating all the waiting is: waiting for referrals, appointments, your period, your ovaries to produce eggs, womb lining to thicken, for egg collection, to find out how many eggs have fertilised, how many develop into embryos, and finally, waiting to discover if you're pregnant.

They share that it's normal and understandable for your emotions to go from one end of the scale to the next in the blink of an eye. And this is OK. It's OK to not be OK. There's so much riding on IVF, and of course, you're going to feel very positive at times, such as when your scan shows your follicles are growing well, to the negative moments, such as when some of your eggs don't fertilise. It's important not to bottle up your feelings and that you find support, however that looks for you. If you aren't already on Instagram, this is a great place to find the support you need at this time in your life. And it's not just for women but for their partner too, as IVF involves two halves of a couple (though not always).

One plus side of IVF is that we get to see our future child when they're only a two-cell embryo or eight cells or sixteen cells. You may have video footage of your future child dividing and developing that you can show them when they're older. Now that is priceless!

I and all the other contributors sincerely hope you find this book helpful. For many, they found writing about their experience really helped them. For me, I found reading their stories helped me all these years later. Please, don't underestimate how infertility and having fertility treatment affects your mental health. This is much more recognised now and there are contributions from fertility experts who cover this area, so, please, be sure to read their supportive words and if you want to connect with them, you can find their details in the 'Resources' section at the end of the book.

Much love

Sheila xx

A letter to someone who hasn't had IVF

Dear Friend,

Firstly, thank you so much for opening this book. It's probably not the sort of book you'd normally read, but, please, read some of it. I think you'll be interested in what others are sharing about their experience of fertility treatments. I hope you don't mind me starting with the boring, but essential part first. Most people are shocked and surprised when they find out that one in eight couples find it challenging to have a baby, and that the World Health Organisation (WHO) recognises infertility as a disease. Yes, a medical condition. For a large percentage of people, the only way that they'll have their longed-for family is through IVF (in-vitro fertilisation) or another fertility treatment.

Over eight million children have been born since the first IVF baby was born in the UK in 1978. Around 2.5 million IVF cycles are carried out every year around the world and this number increases every year. The mother of the first IVF baby had blocked Fallopian tubes, and therefore, the egg and the sperm were never going to meet whilst they tried to get pregnant naturally. IVF is now used for a variety of medical conditions, such as endometriosis, polycystic ovarian syndrome, early menopause, male factor issues, and for many, there is no known cause.

Having IVF isn't a fast process because you have to wait for the woman to have her period, and as a lot of women may only have a couple of periods a year, this can be a long wait. When you start your cycle, the first blood test/scan to egg collection can be around six weeks. And don't forget, by the time people get to have IVF, they've already been trying to get pregnant for at least one year, but for most, it's many more years.

In the UK some people will get IVF on the NHS, but it's dependant on where they live, and they have to tick a lot of boxes before they're accepted. In some countries like the US, the person's health insurance may cover some of the costs, but the majority of people have to fund their IVF cycle themselves.

The chances of being successful through IVF will depend on the age of the woman's eggs and other factors relevant to the woman and her partner, but on average, thirty-seven per cent of IVF cycles for women under thirty-five result in a baby, so sixty-three per cent of cycles aren't successful. The chances of success reduce with age.

Most people will go through more than one IVF cycle. The results of one study were that a couple would have on average 2.7 IVF cycles before they were successful. After three IVF cycles, the odds for success are between thirty-four to forty-two per cent.

IVF involves a lot of medications, blood tests, ultrasound scans of ovaries and womb linings, injections, emotions, tears and money. The process isn't entered into lightly, it takes a very strong person/couple to get through the demands, not only on the woman's body but fitting it into their lives.

Some people will tell others that they're receiving IVF treatment and some keep it to themselves. Often people don't want to worry their family or friends but mostly they keep quiet because if you haven't been through IVF, it's hard to understand exactly what it's like. Inadvertently, people say insensitive things like: "You'll get pregnant now you're having IVF", "You can have my children" or "Just relax." None of these help at all. If someone has told you they're receiving IVF, simply let them know you're there when they need you. Please, don't try and fix their problem. You can't! They have a team of highly trained medical professionals working on 'Project Baby.' Don't be offended if your invites are turned down: appointments, scans, injections must all happen on certain days and sometimes at specific times. And with all the hormones being taken, the woman won't know from one day to the next how she's going to feel emotionally. Please just be there when you are needed. Thank you.

Much love,

Sheila xx

The Grief of IVF

It's not unusual to find yourself grieving before and after an IVF cycle. Your grief is real and should be validated. Just because you can't physically see what you're grieving, doesn't mean you're not grieving.

When we think of grief, it's associated with losing someone close to us, someone who was alive and now isn't, and people accept that we'll be upset and often depressed. But grief, when you're going through IVF, is much harder for another person to understand, because what you're grieving for can't be seen or touched.

Most people who go through IVF are grieving for many different things and as we're all unique, it varies from one person to another. It isn't just the woman who's grieving, her partner will be too. And if she/they have shared their journey with their parents, for example, they may also be grieving that they'll never become grandparents.

They may grieve because they can't get pregnant naturally. They'll never experience wondering when exactly they conceived, the spontaneity around conceiving, that it was only them and their partner involved in the conception and that getting pregnant shouldn't be hard work, it should just happen.

When you start an IVF cycle, whether it's your first or fifth, you won't know the outcome; it isn't guaranteed. After having blood tests, scans, nasal sprays and injections, your body may not respond – you either don't grow any follicles or your womb lining doesn't thicken – so, your cycle is cancelled by the clinic. At the time of this being written, the world is dealing with the Covid-19 pandemic and fertility clinics internationally have stopped all treatments. This means that many have had their egg collections cancelled, despite taking their medications and having blood tests and scans; frozen transfers have also been cancelled, again, despite all the preparation beforehand, or an IVF cycle didn't start when it was due to. Not only is this extremely upsetting, but you may find you're grieving for what could have been.

During IVF you are growing, hopefully, more than one follicle in your ovaries. We are all desperate for each scan to reveal as many follicles as possible because in each follicle we hope there's a good quality, mature egg. All your efforts are focused on follicles and eggs because eggs make babies. You're far more aware of your eggs than someone who falls pregnant naturally because you've imagined them during the scans, maybe heard the embryologist calling out each time an egg is present in the follicle liquid during egg collection/retrieval, so you're their biggest fan. Once egg collection occurs, you're now willing all your eggs to fertilise. As far as you're concerned, each egg is your future child and you're already planning what your life will be like with them in it. Unfortunately, not every egg that's collected fertilises. Even if an egg does fertilise, there's no guarantee that the cells will divide as they should do. Suddenly, you're losing your future children and there's nothing you can do. If this happens, it's natural to feel a tsunami of emotions from sadness and anger to shock and grief.

You may have planned a 'freeze all' cycle with your clinic, which means that any embryos created are frozen, usually on day five, and you'll be prepared for that. However, you may have decided that an embryo will be transferred straight away on day two, day three or day five. You'll expect this to happen and be prepared mentally. But if you develop an emergency condition known as OHSS (ovarian hyperstimulation syndrome – where too many follicles grow), an embryo probably won't be transferred. Any that are of good quality will be frozen for a future cycle. Sadly, none may develop to the required quality. If this happens, it's understandable that you'll grieve for the embryos … your children that haven't made it.

The whole reason for doing IVF is to get pregnant and to have a baby, but it's by no means guaranteed. After an embryo is transferred, there's the 'dreaded' two-week wait, because it's roughly two weeks before you're advised to do a pregnancy test. During this time, you're what is referred to within the

Trying to Conceive community, as 'PUPO' – Pregnant Until Proven Otherwise. You cannot see what's going on inside your womb, so you visualise your embryo snuggling in – you talk to it, stroke your tummy, and build a mother/child relationship, loving it as if it's already born. Remember, if someone falls pregnant naturally, at this point, they don't know that their egg has been fertilised by their partner's sperm and the embryo has implanted, so they can't love their future child yet. But because we know that an embryo was transferred, we're already pouring all our love into our future child. At the end of the two-weeks, if you get a negative pregnancy test, you immediately feel grief-stricken and often shock because your child no longer exists. Unless you have experienced this, it's hard to understand. What we want people to acknowledge is that the bundle of cells that was transferred was our future baby, just as if it had been born nine months later. That baby would have been someone's son or daughter, grandchild, niece or nephew, godchild or sibling. Our loss is real.

Having the support of others in recognising our loss, enables us to address our grief and share our sadness that we don't have children yet. Validating loss can be important for many and makes it easier for us to live with it. There are usually triggering events that bring grief to the surface, such as pregnancy announcements, an invite to a baby shower, holiday times where there'll be babies and children and inevitable questions. To help with the grief, acknowledge to yourself that the situation is likely to cause you upset by understanding why does this event hurt – such as why do people ask questions about when you're going to have children. Often, they're just making conversation or are curious. Think about how you might answer their question – you may be polite, snarky, or just deflect it – it's totally up to you. Instead of saying something to their face, you can always make a retort in your head – which may help to control your emotions.

The most important thing in getting through loss and grief and coming out intact the other side is having hope and support. Research reveals that people who are grieving any sort of loss and can identify hope in the future, move through their sorrow with a better outcome. It may be that right now feeling hopeful is hard; even being optimistic that you'll get out of bed today is enough or that you'll pray tomorrow is better than today. Finding non-judgemental support – wherever that may be – will enable you to express and explore your feelings, because they are as justified as the next persons.

Sheila @fertilitybooks

Imagine if...

You'll have to take medication that won't actually make you feel better

You'll have to inject yourself daily and you're scared of needles

You'll have to inject yourself, hundreds of times over multiple cycles, in the hope you'll get pregnant

You'll have to have tests, investigations, painful procedures, scans, blood tests, injections, operations, maybe all for nothing

You're asked multiple times, over many years, 'when are you having a baby?'

You're told to 'just relax' over and over again for something that's out of your control

You're always waiting

You've spent all your savings and still there's no baby

You've gone into debt and still there's no baby

You've never seen two pink lines or the word 'Pregnant' on a pregnancy test stick

You'll never hear or see your baby's heartbeat at the ultrasound scan

You'll never make the decision whether to find out the sex of your baby at the scan

You'll never make an announcement on social media that you're pregnant

You'll never touch your pregnant belly

You'll never feel your baby move inside you

You'll never shop for the cot, pushchair, high chair, sling, car seat for your baby

You'll never decorate your baby's nursery

You'll never announce the birth of your baby

You'll never introduce your baby to your family and friends

You'll never share with your child their story of how they were conceived

You'll never take your baby's photo with the weekly/monthly milestone board

You'll never feel the warmth or weight of your baby lying on your chest

You'll never buy or dress your baby in that cute Easter bunny/pumpkin/elf/angel/Santa outfit you've seen every year in your favourite store

You'll never bake and decorate your child's birthday cakes

You'll never see the look of delight on your child's face when they see their birthday cakes

You'll never see your child clapping their hands as you sing 'Happy Birthday' to them

You'll never sing your favourite nursery rhyme with your child

You'll never buy them their first pair of shoes

You'll never wake up in bed to find your child's warm body snuggled up next to you

You'll never make snow or sand angels with your child

You'll never see them perform in the school play

You'll never explain to your child about the tooth fairy, and pretend to be the tooth fairy

You'll never make your parents grandparents

You'll never hear your child tell you they love you.

Imagine if you didn't have all your memories of these precious moments of pregnancy or of your child or children.

Imagine what it's like for me, so desperate to experience all that you have, but not knowing if I'll ever have these memories.

Sheila @fertilitybooks

The truth about IVF

Infertility is a medical condition and unlike other illnesses usually affects two people. IVF is a medical procedure as it involves medications, injections, blood tests, scans, surgery and a myriad of emotions. Let me enlarge:

- Consultations with a doctor

- Blood tests to measure hormone levels

- Scans of your ovaries and your womb lining

- Losing your dignity from said scans

- Often minor surgery for endometriosis, fibroids, scar tissue

- The man masturbating, and not for pleasure

- Sniffing a nasal spray

- Injections – hundreds of them if over several cycles

- Bruises from the injections

- Side effects from the medications – bloating, headaches, nausea, mood swings

- Surgery to hopefully collect eggs – it's not always successful

- Hours spent on research

- A massive financial bill causing stress to most

- Tears, anger, sadness, depression, worry, sleepless nights, pain, hurt, hate, envy, lost friendships

- Takes away the spontaneity in your sex life

- A baby is not going to be created through making love

- It's not two people making a baby, instead there's a team:

- Doctors

- Nurses

- Embryologists

- Sonographers

- Pharmacists

- Egg donor (maybe)

- Sperm donor (maybe)

- Embryo donor (maybe)

- Clinic receptionists

- Counsellor

- Coach (maybe)

- Acupuncturist (maybe)

- Nutritionist (maybe)

- Reflexologist and other holistic practitioners (maybe)

- Bank manager (possibly) to pay for this team of skilled professionals and all the home pregnancy tests

- A community of others cheering you on

• Takes over your life; it creeps into every area until you can't remember what your life was like pre-IVF

• It's not guaranteed to be successful

• A lot of patience is needed for all the waiting

• There's no excitement in missing a period and wondering…

• Not being able to surprise your partner with a positive pregnancy test because you both know when test day is

• Makes you extremely anxious when you get a positive pregnancy result.

Sheila @fertilitybooks

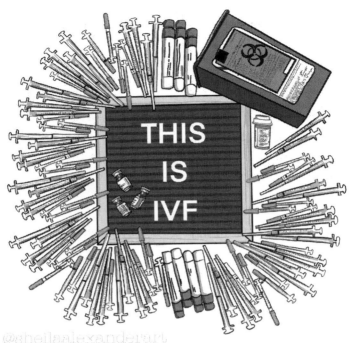

Never apologize

Working through infertility trauma, which includes IVF and fertility treatments, isn't about communication – it's about validation, because it doesn't matter how much we talk about something if we're not truly feeling seen and heard. What we can realize through living life with infertility is that the closest people to us are not always truly able to support us through challenges. We then have to establish how to connect with family and friends, accepting that we're not always able to empathize with each other, and that's okay. Never apologize.

Just because they might not understand, doesn't mean you aren't entitled to time and support.

Never apologize that on some days you can't be optimistic. Never apologize for feeling angry and bitter. Never apologize for putting your dreams of a baby ahead of anything else. Never apologize for taking care of yourself and your health. Never apologize for not being there for others as you grieve or heal. There's no time frame you need to meet. Never apologize for protecting yourself from triggers, even if that means avoiding people you love. Never apologize for not sharing emotionally with everyone, because a) not everyone deserves that part of you, and b) not everyone wants to authentically help or understand. They might just be curious. There's a difference. Don't apologize for how you navigate this new territory.

Please protect your heart whilst you need extra understanding. Most of all protect your raw emotions. Allow yourself time to nourish your soul, pamper, and recharge which connects you back to the things that give you joy and made you feel passionate. You don't have to be there for everyone else and give yourself the leftover scraps. It's okay to be tired and allow yourself rest. Don't apologize or feel guilty for nourishing yourself.

Some friendships won't be able to handle the reality of what you need and what your limits are due to infertility trauma and loss. It's okay to put some relationships on hold. This can be done gently and with love and respect. It's one hundred per cent essential to put your healing before anything or anyone else. You don't have to shrink your pain to make things 'easier' for everyone. Infertility trauma encompasses very similar emotional obstacles and stigmas as chronic illness and PPD (post-partum depression). There's a huge misconception in society that infertility emotions are about 'feeling sad' because you can't get pregnant as fast as you'd hoped. The more we keep highlighting the realities of what infertility is and the trauma involved, the better the understanding and support will be. The more support women get at this crucial stage will only help make any future process an easier transition, whether that be motherhood or something else.

Trying to conceive can be frustrating, scary and lonely at times, especially after numerous attempts. Couples are often left wondering: Why is this happening to us? What are we doing wrong? Where should we go from here? Stress and anxiety can increase with each passing month. Despite the wonderful medical intervention couples receive, the mental and emotional support is often missed in the process. The goal of counselling is to allow you to feel understood and gain the tools to help process fluctuating emotions; to help you explore why you're feeling jealousy, anger or a disconnect to people around you. Ultimately, it's to help you gain insight as you work through any new obstacles that may arise.

Chiemi Rajamahendran @missconceptioncoach

The loss of your embaby

We have words for the loss of a baby, such as miscarriage and stillborn—these terms based ontrimester technicalitiesthat feel clinical and cold. Loss is loss. Pain is pain. Grieving the death of a life that was growing inside of you, a life that could've existedat any stage...there are simply no words. None.

We don't have a word for when someone goes through fertility treatment like IVF or IUI and it 'fails.' The loss of that 'Emby Baby' is just as real, painful and devastating. The added stress of these treatment plans, injections, procedures,and on top of that, the monetary pressure, is unfathomable. Yet it's done unselfishly out of love. Words like chemical pregnancy, blighted ovum, missed pregnancy, all stop us from feeling the connection we have and even the validation we need. They leave us questioning what we'regrievingfor. Was it a real pregnancy? Do I have the right to be sad? Does my loss even matter? It does matter. Say the word 'baby'. Use the word 'grief'. The love for many mothersis instantaneous,from the moment your baby is inside of you.

What do you do with the pain of your hopes and dreams slipping away? People say insensitive things like "you can just try again," but the pain of allowing yourself to be vulnerable again feels like too much. The pain of promising yourself you wouldn't get invested so early, but did, because how could you not? You sit in shock and defeat, ready to give up, not because you want to, but because you can't fathom heartbreak on this level, again. Where does your support come from to get through this loss? Maybe half of the people in your life don't know what you've endured. Most won't understand and you might not want to share such deep personal feelings with others. So, you smilethrough your pain, pretending you're ok. The pain we feel about infertility and grief isn't just about losing what we loved. It's about grieving the moments and experiences we should have had but don't get to.

So, it's ok to be angry and say:

'I should bethe mother of a three-month old now.'

'I was supposed to be twenty weeks pregnant now'.

I know it's not fair and it hurts.

It really, really hurts.No one going through infertility,trauma and loss haveto prove their worthiness or right to grieve. Infertility trauma happened to you, not because of you. You'reprocessing an experience you had no control over. You deserve unconditional support and compassion to help you heal from this loss. Whatever emotions you'reworking through today, just know you'reentitled to them. You'reentitled to have them validated, not questioned. You'reentitled to have them heard, not shamed. You'reentitled to have them held, not dismissed.It's not just a 'failed cycle,' it'sa loss. You have the right to mourn inany way that helps you process and heal.

Chiemi Rajamahendran @missconceptioncoach

IVF is a treatment for infertility, not a luxury

Taken from an Instagram post on 25th June 2019

IVF is NOT simply a choice

NOT a luxury

NOT an opportunity for a 'designer baby'

IVF is a treatment for infertility.

I've had a bee in my bonnet recently, ever since reading some highly insensitive, misinformed comments. The first in response to a fellow blogger's IVF update, followed by some ignorant responses to a celebrity couple announcing the start of their IVF journey. Reading them left me speechless, but have now inspired this post which will hopefully educate a few people along the way! ♥

Some say IVF is a choice – we can choose whether or not we have treatment, that we could "just adopt" or live a life without children. Unbelievably, some say there's divine intervention at play, meaning we weren't meant to become parents. What utter bull!! Sadly, there's no rhyme or reason, we're just unlucky. ♥

IVF is NOT simply a choice, or a luxury, or an opportunity to try for a 'designer baby'. IVF is a treatment for infertility – a disease of the reproductive system recognised by the World Health Organisation. It isn't just an 'elective procedure' as some workplaces consider it. As many as one in six couples are dealing with infertility in the UK, often in silence. ♥

What people with this view haven't considered is that this implied 'choice' becomes impossible as the drive to become a parent cannot be 'switched off.' We've evolved to have a primal instinct to reproduce, a driver engrained so deeply within our brains and society that our emotions don't allow us to simply 'move on.' When we're told we aren't able to reproduce naturally, it's devastating, and so we look for something…

anything… that can help. Thank goodness we live in a generation where we can have treatment to overcome infertility.

When a couple undergoes IVF or other medical treatments to help them get pregnant, it needs to be understood that we're simply doing whatever we can to become parents, which can be sadly taken for granted by those who have no trouble conceiving. Many have no idea how much we'd love to conceive without the emotional, physical and financial turmoil that infertility can bring, often with a detrimental impact on our mental health.

The celebrity couple slated for sharing their story, I'd imagine aren't doing IVF just for a publicity stunt. They're probably devastated they can't conceive naturally like many of us. We should be grateful to them for speaking out, as by doing so they help many of us feel less alone.

Please THINK about your words and how they might impact others. Those experiencing infertility shouldn't have to face the comments I read in complete horror this past week. Empathy is so important in all aspects of life – put yourself in another's shoes, and if you still can't understand, maybe it's better to say nothing at all.

Becky Kearns @definingmum

When IVF fails

When my husband and I tried IVF after eighteen months of unexplained infertility, I remember a feeling of excitement. "This is it", I thought, the help we need to finally start a family. I felt confident it would work for us because we were reasonably young and had no major health issues to overcome. I had no idea what it entailed or how much strength I would need to get through it.

We went through four rounds of IVF before we became pregnant with our daughter, and what surprised me the most was the grief that came with each failed cycle. I was convinced that our first round would work because we had a top-grade embryo transferred and my doctor seemed really confident. I'd prepared myself for success, so the phone call that gave us a negative test result was heart-wrenching. I remember collapsing on the floor in hysterics as my husband tried to lift me up to hug me, and I kept saying: "But it's not fair, this was supposed to work, it was supposed to be our time". The only thing comparable is the loss of a loved one. I sobbed uncontrollably for days, it hit me so hard. I never expected to feel that way and it shocked me. It took a while to get over the devastation that our first failed cycle caused, but after a few months, we were ready to try again with another cycle.

The next one using a frozen embryo created many more hurdles to overcome. I worried our embryos might not survive being thawed, and preparing my body with progesterone had its challenges, as I found it affected my mood more than other hormone medications. We decided to transfer two embryos this time to give ourselves a better chance. Even after our first cycle failed, we felt positive about this one.

Everything went well and we waited patiently for the phone to ring at lunchtime with the results of our blood test. I'll never forget how nervous we were as we stared at the phone, waiting for it to ring. I jumped when it did and knew immediately it was bad news from the tone in the nurse's voice. My husband tried to keep me positive, but I was utterly devastated once again. Another grieving period for the baby we came so close to having. During our two-week wait, I already felt bonded with the baby or babies that were possibly starting to grow inside me. I talked to them, I touched my belly and did everything mentally I could to encourage our embryos to stick around. But we had lost the chance of parenthood yet again.

We picked ourselves up and after a few months prepared for another frozen cycle with two more quality embryos. Third time lucky, I thought. Again, everything went well, and we overcame every hurdle – our embryos survived being thawed, my womb lining was thick enough and the embryo transfer was straight forward. Then there was another stomach-turning moment waiting for the phone to ring and another answer I couldn't bear to hear: "I'm so sorry Suzanne, but your test is negative. My prayers weren't answered today, either," our nurse said, trying to offer some comfort. I felt broken and in utter despair, feeling sad and angry. What was wrong with me? Surely something must have been missed in my investigations? That was the darkest time, having three failed rounds of IVF. I felt like a failure – I couldn't get pregnant naturally nor could I make it work through IVF. Why couldn't I make our embryos stay in my womb and grow?

Just when I thought things couldn't get any worse, the progesterone you take to build the lining of your womb means a heavy bleed will follow. I've always suffered from painful periods, but this was on another level. Even with strong pain relief, the cramps were excruciating. It was like the final straw dealing with this physical pain alongside my mental anguish. I'm sure it's different for everyone but I wish I'd been better prepared as nobody warned me.

The three failed cycles we experienced brought devastation and grief like I'd never experienced. You invest so much in a cycle of IVF and overcome so many hurdles for a small chance of success. If it fails, it's difficult to accept and understand.

Thankfully, our story doesn't end there and after our fourth round of IVF, we heard the words: "Your test is positive". I can't explain how that felt. It made everything worth it! We'd done a few things differently in preparation for this cycle and were over the moon that everything worked out. We had a new doctor and new clinic funded by the NHS, and our doctor instilled us with confidence, giving us brilliant advice on how to prep for our embryo transfer. This enabled us to have a smooth transfer with no issues. I also prepared myself mentally and physically with acupuncture, kinesiology, healthier eating and positive affirmations. I can't pinpoint what made the difference, perhaps it was a combination of everything.

We now have a beautiful daughter, Georgia, and I'm so grateful we eventfully had success through IVF. Unfortunately, it's an unpredictable process and some people are successful the first time, while others try multiple times. I'd encourage anyone going through it to be open, take all the support on offer, and keep hope in your heart. Even a glimmer of it will keep you going.

Suzanne Minnis @thebabygaim

Frozen embryos when your family is complete

Deciding to donate our frozen embryos to science was the hardest thing I've ever had to do in my life. Even writing this is something I've put off as it makes me feel numb and sad and I've been trying to protect myself. What I'm about to write might well trigger you, so please, don't read on if you're feeling vulnerable about where you are on your journey.

The thing is, I know in my heart I wanted to have more than one more child, however, the reality wasn't the case. We had a successful treatment in 2015, and our son Phoenix is now five.

For the last two years, I've been struggling with the decision of what to do with our three frozen embryos whilst being immersed in the TTC community both on and offline. Creating 'The Fertility Podcast' has been therapeutic in many ways, as I've been lucky to speak to a lot of people about different infertility issues we face along the way. Yet, it's also been a challenge for me to continue while making this decision.

Eventually, I sought professional help, and it's something I highly recommend if you're struggling to make decisions. My husband and I both have siblings, and the guilt I have around our son not having a brother or a sister is immense. Only last night I watched a programme on TV where two sisters in their forties were mourning the loss of their mother – together. I felt instantly upset that Phoenix won't have that support when the inevitable happens.

I spoke with a fertility implications counsellor to work through the process of donating our embryos to science. My husband didn't want to talk about anything. This has since changed, ironically. I think something has lifted within him as a result of our decision. I don't want to go into the reasons why we chose not to have further treatment as they're personal, but it was predominantly financial and that makes me sad. A friend said to me: "What if you fell pregnant naturally? You'd cope, right?" The answer is, yes, of course I would, but that wasn't the situation we were in.

If you do donate your embryos to science, you'll have to accept that you'll grieve. You'll feel sad and you'll cry. You'll still get triggered by things you see on social media; pregnant tummy's that you thought didn't bother you will once again be everywhere. But knowing that you're helping someone else is the one saving grace in this difficult, almost impossible, decision. Someone said to me: "You need to be one hundred percent certain before you do it" – yet, I still wasn't, after two years of thinking about it.

When you tell your clinic that this is what you want to do, there's paperwork to deal with, then more paperwork asking you if you're really sure. It's heartbreaking all over again.

When we finally sent the letter back to the clinic, I wanted to mark the occasion with my husband. We went to the beach and cast three white roses out to sea. Of course, they came back to us, floating on a wave as if to say – hang on, we're still here ... So, I left them in the sand and walked away with tears, once again, rolling down my face. As I turned to look back, I saw a lady with her family stop and crouch down. She was taking photos of the flowers. Just like the embryos going to science to help others, I knew that beautiful image of the roses on the sand was going to bring her joy. It probably made a lovely Instagram shot. It certainly did on my feed.

I have since been back to my clinic and talked about our decision to donate our embryos with their Head of Science, who told me what a gift it is for everyone involved in embryo research, as they are so precious. And for that, I feel really proud of what we have done.

If you want to talk more about this issue, please do get in touch.

Natalie Silverman @fertilitypoddy

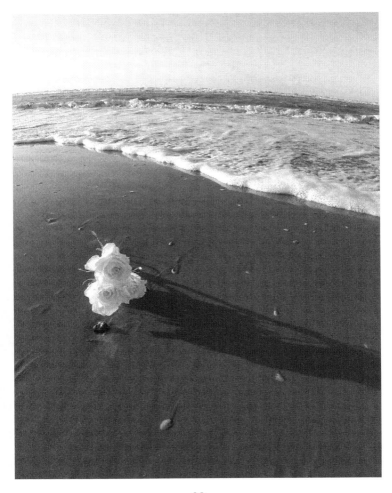

Juggling IVF and your job

I didn't consciously recognise that trying to conceive was affecting me at work until I bumped into a *very* pregnant colleague in the toilets one day. I came out of the cubicle whilst she was washing her hands. I hadn't seen her for months, and there she was – seven or eight months pregnant. She said "Hello" then left the toilets, and I turned around, went back into the cubicle and sobbed and sobbed until there were no tears left. That was over four years ago, and yet, I still remember what she was wearing and more importantly, how I felt such a failure. Before then, I approached our 'trying' with the logic that sooner or later it would happen to us. Everyone around me seemed to get pregnant with no problems, and I'd just had one of my team leave for maternity leave for the third time. The THIRD time, and admittedly, I felt jealous that it happened so easily for her.

When we were finally told IVF was our only viable option, I didn't think to let my boss know as it was private, and nothing to do with work – and to be honest, I didn't have a clue what it would involve. I look back now and see how naïve I was, and sad that there wasn't any support in place. Most people who need a doctor or hospital appointments for a medical condition work them around their job, and that's exactly what myself and my husband did. He took some of his annual leave when we attended appointments or worked split shifts, often meaning he'd start at 7 a.m. and work until 10 p.m. I, too, moved heaven and earth to ensure I wouldn't inconvenience work when ironically, *we* were the ones that needed support.

It was after our second failed IVF cycle that we took a break and reflected on how to manage our third and *last* try. Again, our jobs weren't something we discussed and this time it would be a bigger challenge as the clinic we chose for our treatment was based in London, which meant no more 'nipping out' for appointments, given it was a two-hour train journey from where we lived.

I'm very relieved we didn't consider our jobs when deciding on the right clinic for us, as our third IVF cycle was a success. Our employers were thankfully led by what we needed. I worked on the train to and from London for most appointments – if I was able – as I needed to show my boss I was still doing a good job. I wish now I'd asked for more support from a work perspective, as I dictated ninety-nine per cent of what happened during the cycle, because like thousands of organisations, there was no management or best practice guidance to refer to.

It was after our daughter was born that I reflected on this part of our journey as well as the millions of people worldwide who face the same challenges. I talked to many who'd also held down a job whilst going through IVF and asked them what their employers had done for them. Turns out, not much! The fact that men and women are working as normal whilst juggling infertility treatment isn't on the corporate radar, which is incredibly sad when there's clearly a need for it. Some lost their jobs due to treatment and others felt they couldn't continue due to the stress it put on them and their relationships. I felt really angry about it. Infertility and fertility treatment don't seem to be an important enough issue for organisations to recognise the impact it has on their workforces' wellbeing. It seems a common theme that if you have a supportive line manager, even in the absence of official guidance, then everything will be less stressful, but as fertility treatment doesn't often go to plan, even this isn't always a given.

My top tips for managing work around fertility treatment are:

- Be honest from the beginning with your employer as this supports anything that follows. In the absence of any management guidance or policy for fertility treatment, then think carefully about what is 'reasonable' for both the business and you to commit to. Going through fertility treatment is stressful enough without having pressure from work too.

- Depending on your role, are you able to work flexibly during treatment? This could mean working remotely or from home. Asking for the means to do this is reasonable, such as a laptop and/or phone if you work for a larger organisation. For smaller companies, work collaboratively with your employer to decide what this may look like for you.

- Understand your treatment and what happens when, so you know when you'll be unable to work, i.e. after egg collection. If annual leave is suggested try and negotiate *some*, not *all* of it being taken this way, as your annual leave/holidays are for relaxation, not to recover from a medical procedure.

It's not all doom and gloom. I've heard about 'exceptionally supportive' line managers who listened to what their employees needed by allowing them to work from home, and even reduced workloads temporarily to alleviate the pressure. Some have even been allowed paid time off for treatment. The most supportive measure I've heard of is how an employer allowed their employee to work the whole two-week wait from home for the minimum amount of stress.

A lot of people battle secretly doing IVF or other fertility treatments whilst continuing to work 'normally', and you never know where you're going to find a kindred spirit as many more people are affected by infertility than you think. The corporate world is changing and the more everyone can bang this drum to make changes for the future, the better. If you're in a privileged position where you can influence your organisation, I hope that reading this gives some insight into what's needed.

Claire Ingle @ivfatwork and @fertilitymattersatwork

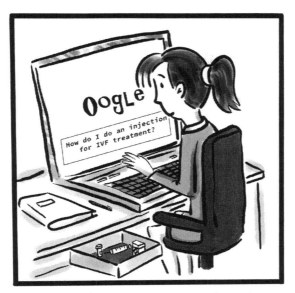

Doing IVF when working – most people
have chocolate in their desk drawer...

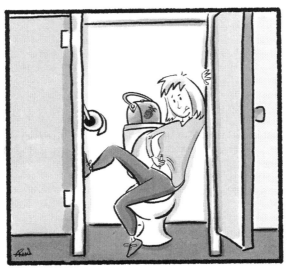

Sometimes you have no choice where you do the
injections – today, the toilet at work...

Why male fertility tests are important

For some reason, I've always thought I'd struggle to have children. I can't explain why. Maybe it's my mindset, always preparing for the worst-case scenario. Hence, I was kind of prepared. It was still very upsetting, but we were positive with every cycle. We really believed it was going to work.

I've complained to the NHS (UK) as I was given a basic semen analysis and that was it. After three rounds of ICSI (intracytoplasmic sperm injection) on the NHS, I went privately for tests. Before the appointment, I was told to do more tests: Sperm Comet, (a test to find out if there's any DNA fragmentation in the sperm), hormone, sperm neutral, urine, oxidative stress, and probably a few more that I've forgotten. Unsurprisingly, the NHS weren't interested in any of these tests and continued with our fertility treatment, even when the DNA fragmentation test confirmed I had DNA damage high enough to be linked to infertility. So ICSI was unlikely to be successful. Fertilisation always occurred but several miscarriages suggested issues with the sperm quality.

I felt completely left out during appointments. I remember the consultant saying we only need one good sperm. At no point did anyone ever mention the quality of what was contained within the sperm. They even told me, as fertilisation always occurred, that this suggested nothing was wrong with the sperm – which was false – but they also told me my wife's egg would repair any DNA damage. I've since been told by a leading expert in the field that this was also completely wrong due to my wife's age.

Gareth James, UK

The importance of genetic testing

"I'm sorry — she's gone." Those are the words that torment me. Spoken to me the moment after my daughter took her last breath.

On 11 March 2017, my husband Jonathan and I welcomed our beautiful daughter, Mackenzie into the world. Mackenzie was extremely loved. A beautiful blonde-haired baby with big expressive blue eyes and the most beautiful coo.

After Mackenzie was born, we were in a bubble of bliss. She was perfect. However, at ten weeks of age, a routine lactation consult started a series of events that changed our world forever. The lactation consultant commented that Mackenzie should be moving more. What followed in the next two days was a doctor's appointment, a paediatrician appointment, and a neurologist appointment culminating in devastating news. At ten weeks of age, Mackenzie was diagnosed with a genetic illness called spinal muscular atrophy (SMA) type 1. We were told it was terminal and Mackenzie only had months to live. At that moment, the image of our future smashed to pieces, along with our hearts.

SMA type 1 or Werdnig-Hoffmann disease is a form of motor neuron disease affecting the lower motor neurons in the spinal cord. When they stop sending messages properly to the muscles, the affected person loses the ability to move and their muscles slowly waste away due to inactivity. The muscles closest to the trunk are the first to be affected, including the upper arms, shoulders, hips, back and upper legs. Next, the person struggles to swallow, making eating difficult. They have difficulty coughing and cannot shift any mucus from their chest, so colds are a serious issue that can lead to life-threatening pneumonia. Eventually, they lose the ability to breathe, becoming trapped inside their bodies.

Amongst all the emotions, the pain and devastation, we asked ourselves: "How did this happen?" Mackenzie was a planned baby. We'd done every single test available to us to check our health before pregnancy, during pregnancy and post-birth, including the non-invasive parental test (NIPT) which looks at chromosomal issues such as Down Syndrome, and the newborn screen test (otherwise known as the heel prick test). Every test revealed we had a healthy baby girl to love.

We discovered that SMA is a genetic condition. A genetic condition is a disorder that's caused by an abnormality in an individual's DNA. Specifically, SMA is a recessive genetic condition, meaning both Jonathan and I are carriers.

Although some genetic conditions can be caused by a gene mutation, most genetic disorders are hereditary. It takes two defective genes, one from the mother and one from the father, which sits in their DNA and can be passed on to potential children. When two people carry the same condition, they have a twenty-five per cent chance of having an affected child, a twenty-five per cent chance of having an unaffected child, and a fifty per cent chance of having a child who'd also be a carrier of the condition.

There are also other ways for genetic disorders to be passed on but they are much less common. For example, some conditions are called 'X-linked dominant,' meaning the condition is carried by the mother and passed on to children through her DNA only.

There are thousands of genetic conditions, some rarer than others. When we looked into this, we discovered that on average, every single person carries three genetic conditions in their DNA, and it's down to luck and who they have children with that determines if their child will be born with that condition.

We learnt that there's a simple mouth swab or blood test that can tell you what genetic conditions you carry. If you and your partner both do the test, you can discover what your chances of having an affected child is. This is called a 'genetic reproductive carrier test'. While this test exists already, it costs money and most medical professionals only offer it to those who have a family history. However, studies show that four out of five children born with a genetic condition have no family history, so this practice is flawed and dangerous.

On finding this out, our family campaigned the Australian Government for a genetic reproductive carrier test to be offered routinely and free for all Australians who wanted it. This led to a twenty million-dollar research project called "Mackenzie's Mission" – our daughter's legacy. We hope that in 2022, Mackenzie's Mission will lead to routinely offered free genetic reproductive carrier testing before conceiving, or in early pregnancy.

During our campaigning, the Royal Australian and New Zealand College of Obstetricians and Gynaecologists changed its previous stance to now recommend: 'Information on carrier screening for other genetic conditions should be offered to all women planning a pregnancy or in the first trimester of pregnancy. Options for carrier screening include screening with a panel for a limited selection of the most frequent conditions, e.g. cystic fibrosis, spinal muscular atrophy and fragile X syndrome, or screening with an expanded panel that contains many hundreds of disorders.'

After losing Mackenzie our world fell apart. She was and continues to be our everything. She made us parents and we knew we wanted more children. For people like us who are at risk of having affected children, there are several options including in utero testing where couples get pregnant naturally, then have a test called 'chorionic villus sampling' (CVS), which takes a sample of placental tissue. Or there's an amniocentesis test which takes a sample of the amniotic fluid that surrounds the unborn baby. These tests can show whether a baby has a genetic or chromosomal disorder, and depending on the results, a decision can be made on whether to continue with the pregnancy or have a medical interruption. This is a very scary option and people will feel differently depending on their beliefs, but for some people, this is the only way to have a healthy child who won't be born just to pass away, or to live in pain with a severe and chronic illness. Other options can include sperm, egg or embryo donation.

Finally, there is in-vitro fertilisation (IVF) to ensure a baby doesn't possess the possible genetic condition. In IVF, a fertility specialist can test embryos for particular genetic conditions, so only healthy, unaffected embryos will be implanted in the uterus which is called 'preimplantation genetic diagnosis' (PGD*).

For PGD, couples use IVF to create embryos. The difference is that in 'normal IVF,' embryos are transferred after fertilisation before or on day five. However, for PGD, the process continues to day six, where they hope that the blastocyst will turn into a hatching blastocyst, which means it breaks out of its 'shell' in preparation for implanting on the uterine wall. This hatching is necessary for PGD because this is when the cells are exposed enough for an embryologist to carefully extract a couple of cells which will eventually become the placenta.

The cells are then analysed and within two weeks, you'll be told whether the embryos have the genetic condition they're being tested for. This can also be done in conjunction with 'pre-implantation genetic screening' (PGS*), which tests the embryos for chromosome abnormalities using the same cells extracted for PGD testing.

We're now doing IVF with PGD and PGS in order to have healthy siblings for Mackenzie. We miss our darling daughter more than words will ever describe. Our little shooting star shone fast, but bright, and because of her, Mackenzie's Mission will impact the world.

We believe genetic reproductive carrier testing should be the number one test conducted in order to have a healthy child.

* PGD and PGS were the terms used prior to 2019, nowadays this testing is known as 'Preimplantation Genetic Testing' or PGT, and there are three categories; PGT-A, PGT-M and PGT-SR.

Rachael Casella @mylifeof_love

Unconsciously uncoupling?

It should be one of the best times in a relationship – after all, what could be more romantic and life-affirming than starting a family with the person we love? And yet, for so many couples trying to conceive without success, those initial feelings of physical intimacy and emotional closeness often give way, over the frustrating months and years, to feelings of estrangement and feeling 'lonely together,' as one of my clients recently described it. And it's often at this stage in the journey that couples consider IVF or other methods of assisted reproduction.

Whilst most report some respite from these feelings, unfortunately, research shows that with each unsuccessful cycle of treatment, a couples' distress levels increase. A study commissioned by Fertility Network UK (2016), revealed that ninety per cent of participants described themselves as depressed, and sadly, forty-two per cent, suicidal. More than two-thirds stated that infertility and unsuccessful treatment also had a detrimental impact on the quality of their relationship with fifteen per cent reporting considerable strain or thoughts of ending their relationship.

And whilst the saying goes: 'what doesn't break us, makes us stronger', what I observe in couples coming for therapy is a process I call 'unconscious uncoupling'. A slow and painful sense of emotional drift and estrangement.

And whilst the reasons for this process are often complex, they may include:

- Differences in coping strategies – where one person reaches out for support, the other, feeling overwhelmed, shuts down emotionally.

- Loss of the 'secure base' of the couple's relationship – when the partner can no longer soothe or protect in the way they may have done previously.

49

- Cumulative fertility trauma and pregnancy losses mean the couple turn away from each other to cope.

- Intensity of feelings such as anger or despair may overwhelm the couple, and the fight-flight-freeze response to events becomes the norm in order to survive ongoing fertility treatment.

- Repeated failed cycles may lead to hopelessness and 'learned helplessness' deadening the relationship.

So, what helps?

- Social support in the form of online forums and social media accounts, as well as real-life support from family and friends if the couple are to survive the fertility rollercoaster.

- 'Fertility-free' days when the couple agrees not to engage with fertility issues can offer respite, too.

- Keeping up with shared interests and hobbies may allow for vital 'moments of meeting'.

- It's crucial that couples understand that seeking support outside of the relationship is healthy, and in fact, may lead to greater individual resilience.

- Finding new coping strategies is also important, e.g. grounding techniques, yoga and exercise can help manage the physical impact of stress and anxiety.

- Finally, couples therapy can offer a supportive environment, too.

Julianne Boutaleb @Parenthoodinmind

Was it because of the IVF?

An excerpt from the book *21 Miles: swimming in search of the meaning of motherhood* by Jessica Hepburn

Was it because of the IVF, like Fiona said?

Or did it start before that?

Was it because I made you leave the life you had

to be with me?

Or because I blamed you for the life I left behind

for you?

Was it because I wanted to have a baby?

Was it because I wanted to have a baby more

than you did?

Was it because I went on and on about it until

you looked at me across the dinner table

and agreed?

But then I couldn't. Was it because of that?

Was it because of the IVF?

The indignity.

The actuation of blame.

The debt.

Was it because I wrote a book about it?

Took my tights off for the Daily Mail.

Let Radio 4 come over to our house.

Was it because of that scene you said I'd
    embellished? The one where we have a row
    because you've come home drunk the day
    before our embryos go back.

Was it because I always thought you drank more
    than you said you did?

Insisted on smelling your breath?

Was it because I could never trust you?

About anything.

Wanted to see your texts and emails.

Never believed what you said to me was true.

Was it because I'm too controlling?

Because I always want my own way.

Was it because I hated it when you wore that
    leather jacket that I thought made you
    look old?

Or the time you booked five different restaurants
    as a surprise for my birthday to be sure there
    was one that I liked and I didn't want to go to
    any of them?

Was it because I sometimes got angry and
    threw stuff?

Was it because I threw your favourite book, the

one that you said was really valuable, and it

ripped. Was it because of that?

Was it because we stopped having sex for fun?

Because sex became just about having a baby?

Was it because I became completely obsessed

with having a baby?

And when it didn't happen, I became obsessed

with other things instead.

First work, then writing a book, and then

swimming the Channel.

Was it because I insisted I had to do

something big?

Was it because I did it to heal me, and didn't

think about how to heal you?

Was it all this stuff I did to you?

Or was it the stuff you did to me?

Because you did stuff too.

You did.

Jessica Hepburn @jessica_hepburn_

Accepting that fertility treatment is the only way to have a baby

I believe acceptance is a gift that you give yourself – meaning, you can choose to feel okay about having fertility treatment, rather than continually thinking it wasn't how you imagined becoming a mother would be. When you do this, you're committing to your emotional wellbeing and happiness, acknowledging that your fertility struggle shouldn't be creating upset in your life. You deserve that, don't you? There are important steps you can take that will help with this, so let's look at these.

Sometimes a client will come to me, adamant they don't want to go down the road of fertility treatment to get pregnant. There are many reasons why they feel so strongly, but outside of religious beliefs, their decision can be driven by fear. Fear of possible consequences toward their health, fear of failure, fear of it costing way more than they anticipated, fear of spending all that money and not getting a positive result, fear of the process itself and so on.

From my experience of working with clients since 2007, deciding to have fertility treatment is less about acceptance and more about feeling in control of the decision-making process. When we're fearful we are in an 'Emergency State' and our ability to make good decisions is severely compromised. These fears, of course, don't just come up for those who don't want fertility treatment. Those of you who feel OK about having fertility treatment will also have these fears. So, the following is useful for everybody.

Get out of the 'Emergency State'

The first thing a Freedom Fertility Formula Specialist will do with their clients is help them get out of the 'Emergency State' that they're undoubtedly living in. When a person is living in a high-stress situation, of which in(fertility) is right up there, it sends the message to the ancient part of their brain, which I call the 'Feeling Brain', that they're in actual physical danger. In making good decisions for ourselves, there are three problems with that:

1. In times of stress, the cerebral cortex or the 'Thinking Brain' as I call it, can be emotionally hijacked by the 'Feeling Brain', and we move into reactionary decision making, rather than well thought out decisions using a combination of facts and feelings (more on this in a bit).

2. When a person is in an 'Emergency State', they'll automatically follow those in authority – most likely the advice of their medical caregivers, which is not, in essence, a problem. Doing so, however, without full understanding about why they're being advised to take a course of action, can make them feel pulled along in the process. Making decisions because they've been told to, not necessarily because they feel right.

3. To make matters worse, when we're stuck in an 'Emergency State,' our 'Feeling Brain' automatically seeks to predict the future, at least in the short term. A future based on fear.

Can you see the collective problem with this?

You can, therefore, FEEL hugely out of control. When we move out of the 'Emergency State', we're instead in what I call, a 'Neutral State', in which we're able to use both our 'Thinking' and 'Feeling' brain to make informed decisions.

Making Informed Decisions

When a person is in a 'Neutral State' they use their 'Thinking Brain' to gather facts, and with those facts carry out some analysis around what feels right. Notice I say, "what FEELS right". I don't want to come across all woo-woo, but it's important to appreciate that we're all able to instinctively tune in to what is right for us. I'm sure you've experienced times when you feel that something is 'good' and when you feel like something is 'off'. When we do this, we're using our 'Thinking' and 'Feeling' parts of our brain to make the right decisions for us.

The secret as to whether fertility treatment is the right approach for you is to reclaim emotional control right at the beginning – to make informed decisions, which in turn leads you to the right choice in how to have a baby. Acceptance is then able to follow.

Dany Griffiths @freedomfertilityformula

Our fertility treatment story

My husband and I have been TTC (trying to conceive), since we got married in May 2014. After a year or so of unsuccessful results, all BFN's (negative pregnancy tests), we decided it was time to speak with someone in the medical profession. As much as we didn't like to admit it, we clearly had an 'issue' with getting pregnant naturally.

Months turned into years, with doctor appointments and endless tests - including the horrid HSG (Hysterosalpingogram) test, which was really painful and thirty minutes of raw hell. We finally got the referral for NHS funded cycles: 1x IUI (intra-uterine insemination) and 1x IVF (in vitro fertilisation). We met all the criteria straightaway, so choosing our preferred clinic and getting an appointment with the consultant all happened pretty quickly.

I was put on Clomid for five days and a few scans later, I did the trigger injection and we were in the treatment room having IUI. Unfortunately, this was unsuccessful which baffled me and my husband – why didn't it work? I may have a low egg count but the whole procedure of artificial insemination at the 'right' time meant it shouldn't have failed. Annoyed, we picked ourselves back up and went in for a follow-up appointment. I wanted to try another IUI, self-funded this time, however, the consultant advised it was better to go straight into a cycle of IVF.

I remember us sitting in the room where the consultant was going through the stages of IVF – seeing the little coloured flip diagram of a cartoon uterus and what happens at egg collection made me cringe a little. That needle goes where exactly!? It looked like it went diagonal from my cervix! Laughing nervously, I nodded, as if I knew what to expect. I think I heard the words 'sedation' somewhere, too.

We were put on a long protocol of down-regulation and stimulating injections over a four to five-week period. The first lot of injections were once a day to stop follicles from developing in my ovaries, and during this, I had a bleed as expected. The injections stung, so this was a big challenge for me, mentally and physically, especially since I'm afraid of needles! I wanted to do all the injections myself as it was the only part of this journey where I felt in control. My dear husband was on standby if I needed any help. He was really good like that. I guess he felt guilty I was going through this, yet, I reassured him, we were doing this together.

After our down regs scan, we were given the go-ahead to start stimulation injections, which meant I had to inject three different medications every day. The thought of doing one injection a day was hard, but three was a definite big step! Somehow, through the tears and overthinking, day by day, I made myself inject. It gave me a massive sense of achievement. I never thought I'd do it; it's been a challenging journey, mentally and physically. One good tip I learnt was to keep calm (where possible), clear the mind and use an ice pack prior to injecting.

After thirteen days of stims and three scans of my womb lining later, we were ready to do the trigger injection for egg collection! My scans showed we had about eight follicles. This was a pretty good number for me (with our IUI cycle I only had four follicles), so I felt quite positive.

The morning of egg collection, there was a nervous excitement. Not knowing the outcome was the worse feeling. My husband was called in to work his magic while I was getting ready to go into the treatment room. By this point, my nerves were maxed out! Luckily the staff at the clinic were so comforting, and moments before being sedated, I had a sense of being in good hands. I woke up tired and drowsy with no pain, so I was relieved that I was knocked out from the sedation drugs. A couple of hours later I was fine to leave the clinic and rest at home. The only discomfort was from that awful cannula and slight cramping in my uterus. I took painkillers for the rest of the day.

Our updates post egg collection were good: seven eggs collected and six fertilised which were dividing as they should be. On day three, we had the call to confirm transfer will happen on day five. All six were still dividing nicely.

Day two, post egg collection, I started progesterone capsules, inserted with an applicator into my vagina. I didn't have any problems with this. I must admit, I preferred these rather than the progesterone in oil (POI) injections. Jesus, I think they would have been the ultimate test! I so admire women who go through PIO shots, big up to them!

Transfer day came quickly – my bladder was full as advised. It soon became quite uncomfortable to walk. As we entered the treatment room, the embryologist gave us an update since egg retrieval day. We had two top-grade embryos at the blastocyst stage, but unfortunately, the other four hadn't grown as much, and so they were discarded. My heart sank a little on hearing we lost four embryos, but I had to keep positive with the two we had. One was frozen and the other was transferred back. The procedure was pretty straightforward, same as an IUI where they insert the embryo via a catheter and ultrasound. We were back home in no time and I took a couple of days off work to rest.

I religiously ate pineapple core, drank pomegranate juice, ate brazil nuts and boiled eggs. I wanted to do anything that would help aid implantation and top up the nutrition in my body. The first-week, post-transfer day, I had cramps and felt tired with hot flushes and sore boobs. Could this be it? Or was it the progesterone? I didn't care much as long as I was feeling 'something', better than feeling nothing, right?

The second week, my symptoms seemed to have eased off towards the end of our TWW (two-week wait). By this point, I told myself it had failed. My OTD (pregnancy test day) happened on the Monday. I wasn't excited to test, even though I'd managed to not test during my TWW. I thought OTD was going to be great. I tested. It was a BFN. The first thing I said to my husband was "sorry, it didn't work". He dusted my comments off and said it was 'down to us, not just you,' and even though it was negative it wasn't the be-all and end-all. We could try again. I rang the clinic and they wanted me to do another test the next day, just to be sure, as I hadn't had my period yet. The next day came, and I tested BFN. By the late afternoon, AF (aunt flo - menstrual period) showed up as well. That sealed it!

I felt gutted it hadn't worked but was eager to know about our one frozen embryo. We managed to get a cancelled appointment, so were happy about seeing the consultant soon instead of having to wait for months. By the end of the week, on my way home, all the feelings I should have felt on the Monday (OTD) came flooding out of me, and I cried and cried. Something I needed to do, but I guess it's easier to put on a brave face.

Our follow up appointment was productive, so my positive vibes returned. The consultant advised continuing with a frozen embryo transfer (FET). I had to wait for another cycle of AF, then ring the clinic on day one, and start injections on day twenty-one of that cycle. So, before we started again, we had time for a break – to go out and not worry about injections and timings, to carry on eating well and enjoy our time together again.

It wasn't long before our FET protocol was sent to us and the meds were delivered. It's all happening again – nervousness and excitement were setting in.

Today is CD17, and I start my injections in four days. Who knows where this chapter will take us? All I can say is that with the amazing support from my husband, family and friends, and the TTC community on my Instagram page, I feel blessed to follow other people's journeys and to share ours. It's what it's all about.

@mrandmrsivf

The Embryologists Call

Have I got enough signal?
Quickly, call my phone and check it's working...
Mum?! Can't talk now, hang up hang up!
I think I should charge the battery...
What time did they say they would call?
No, don't go to the loo now, there's no time!
Is the call volume high enough? Just going to check it again..
Signals still good...although I think the reception is better if we go downstairs...
WAIT... it's them!!
I won't pick up on the first ring.. don't want to seem too keen...
Hello?

@fertilitady

Going it alone

IVF's a rough ride. An emotional rollercoaster full of hope, uncertainty, surprises and setbacks. That's the case whatever your circumstances, but it can be particularly challenging going through it alone.

I'm a 'single mother by choice' or 'SMBC' (well, soon to be). One of a growing number of women who've chosen to go it alone and have a baby without a partner. As I write this, I'm fourteen weeks pregnant following a four-year struggle with infertility, which included three rounds of egg freezing, two rounds of IVF, and eventually a successful cycle using both sperm and egg donors. It's been incredibly hard, and I've drawn on reserves of resilience and determination that I didn't know I had. I've also, at times, felt acutely lonely, and I know that feeling is by no means exclusive to solo mums. Fertility struggles can leave us all feeling left out, miserable and misunderstood.

Whether I've felt lonelier than someone going through IVF with a partner is impossible to say. IVF is gruelling and relentless, and I lost count long ago of all the appointments, calls, consultations, scans, injections, pills, pessaries, and blood tests. Having company through it all would have been wonderful, I'm sure. Someone to help take in all the information and advice and work out the best way forward. Someone to turn to when I messed up a drug dose and wasn't sure what to do. Or to help with the injections so I didn't have to turn myself into a contortionist. Someone to cry with when it didn't work, and to celebrate with when it finally did. And someone to help pay the bills! That said, I know being by myself has also had its upsides. I've been able to call all the shots. I've never had to compromise or consider someone else's needs and feelings. I've never felt guilty for not being able to have a child or frustrated with a partner that can't understand my point of view. I've been totally in control – well, as much as anyone can be through IVF – and I've felt fortunate in that.

Often, because I've chosen to do this by myself, I feel I have to get on with it – that it's unfair of me to turn to others for help. But sometimes, it's also felt important to go it alone as if practicing for things to come. I went to each pregnancy blood test alone, waited tensely for the results call, and experienced the devastation of two negatives, and then ultimately the elation of a positive as I stood alone on the streets of Marylebone, London. I went to my first pregnancy scans alone, too. I'm learning, though, that most people like to be asked if they can help – they like to feel valued and able to give support. So, I have reached out quite a bit since – I've had friends and family help me in the final stages of selecting donors, drive me home after I've been sedated for egg collections, and come with me to appointments, scans and transfers.

Throughout the IVF process, I've been aware that as a single woman I'm in the minority, albeit a growing one. There's been lots of little things along the way that hit a nerve – such as every time someone assumed I was a 'Mrs'. The voicemail from the clinic giving instructions on when my partner should provide his sperm sample. The doctor who suggested I discuss options with my husband. The sonographer at my 12-week scan who asked if there was anyone with me – "No, just me" was my response. Small things, but they did sting, especially as emotions ran high through IVF as did my hormones and stress levels. I've learned in all this to steel myself and remember that nobody means to offend.

Finding people who 'get' what I'm going through has been invaluable. For me, these three sources of support have been especially helpful:

Social media

About a year after I started trying for a baby, I reconnected with an old friend after stumbling across her Instagram account. She'd been sharing her experience of going through IVF, and when we chatted, she suggested I might do the same. I set up an account, mainly as a sort of scrapbook for myself, to capture all the little things that happen along the way – the decisions, delays, disappointments and various amusing moments, such as being prescribed Viagra, or realising where all those progesterone pessaries have to go. I hadn't expected to find an entire community of women supporting each other. Women struggling to conceive and undergoing IVF (some at the same clinic as me), fellow solo mums and women who've turned to donors to create their families. There are some great fertility-related groups on Instagram and also on Facebook where I've found support, advice, reassurance, companionship, and a reminder that I'm not alone in this.

Donor Conception Network (in the UK)

I found while there were many people on social media struggling to conceive or going through fertility treatment, it was rare to come across people in my situation – single women like me who'd ended up going down the double donor route. The Donor Conception Network (DCN) in the UK, provides a wealth of information for anyone considering any sort of donor treatment and organises meetups to connect local people in similar situations. The friends I've made through the DCN have been a great source of support and comfort and will continue to be, I'm sure.

Therapy

Something I've found challenging about trying to have a baby by myself is that nobody cares as much as I do. Nobody is as emotionally, physically or financially invested. Lots of people care a great deal, but there isn't someone with me every step of the way who I can rely on ... to talk through everything that happens. Seeing a therapist regularly has helped fill that gap, providing an objective listener to help make sense of my feelings, deal with my frustrations and make decisions about the future. Finding the right person can be a bit of trial and error, but it's well worth it.

Infertility can be a lonely experience whether you're going it alone or not. It's easy to think that the worries I have are down to me being a solo mum, but I've learned that often they're just the doubts that everyone has when they're trying to conceive or expecting a baby – such as: Will I be a good mum? Can I afford it? Am I selfish to want this? How will I cope? I swing from feeling proud and confident to worrying about whether I've made the right choices – for me, but also more importantly for my future child. I'm not alone in that, though. There are lots of us in the same boat and reaching out can make all the difference.

Jocelyn @motheringsolo

Sharing my advice on doing IVF treatment

So, you've had lots of sex and still not made a baby. You've been to your GP for blood tests. Your partner has had his sperm analysed. And now, either privately or via the NHS (UK), you've arrived on the doorstep of the fertility clinic, ready to embark on the emotional rollercoaster that is IVF (in vitro fertilisation).

Unlike most people who have twelve chances (more or less) a year to make a baby, the stakes (and not to mention the cost), are much higher in this offspring lottery.

Our desperation for a baby meant that we couldn't cope with the long wait for NHS treatment, so we decided to go privately. When choosing a private fertility clinic, you must shop around. You're spending a not so insubstantial amount of money, and will be trusting them with your most precious embryos; it has to feel right. Go to lots of open days, check the HFEA website (in the UK) for success rates, ask around for recommendations and get all your questions answered. The nurses and doctors are your baby making team; they'll be delivering hopefully good news, but often bad too, so a clinic with compassion is a must.

Make sure you're as emotionally ready as you can be. That may seem like silly advice, as you're about to undergo what can be a hugely stressful period of your life, but self-care is a priority. It could be meditation, acupuncture, walking in nature or baking, it doesn't matter. Also, set aside time for you and your partner and keep talking to each other.

Figure out how you're going to work the treatment schedule around your work. IVF involves daily, or alternate day, scans and blood tests. During my first round of IVF, I kept working and I went back to work in the afternoon after having my embryo transfer in the morning! At the time it felt right, as I was glad of the distraction and I hadn't wanted to make a fuss at work. We're about to embark on our second cycle and I'm taking the entire time off, so I can devote all my energy and focus on making more good embryos.

Now is the time to get over any fear of needles you may have, because the injections and the blood tests will come thick and fast. Many people trust their partner with the injections as a way of keeping them involved. Personally, I'm a control freak, and as a midwife I'm used to giving injections, therefore my husband wasn't allowed anywhere near them! I gave myself a little reward, usually a square of dark chocolate after each injection, and setting an alarm on my phone meant that I wouldn't forget to do them.

Please don't compare your body's response to the drugs with anyone else's. Yes, they may have made thirty-two follicles and you're growing a steady three, but actually what use is thirty-two if none have an egg that goes on to make a good embryo? Everyone's journey is different, and sometimes it's important to focus on your own path. IVF is very dynamic and how you respond to the drugs can change very quickly. I remember crying on my acupuncturist's couch because only one follicle was growing. Then at my scan two days later there were three more, and on egg collection day we ended up with a few more; it's not over until it's over.

Breaking the process down into small chunks made it far more manageable. Each part of the cycle has its own complexities so try not to look too far ahead; take one day at a time. As much of the treatment is out of our control, I needed to regain it in other areas of my life. I did this by eating as well as I could and making sure my head was as clear as possible. Think about what you could do.

And finally, I have to mention progesterone, or as I call them, bum bullets. As a midwife, I have no shame in talking about topics like this. I started taking the pessaries vaginally and ruined several pairs of knickers and disliked the oily feeling. The only way is to do them rectally. Once you've gotten over your squeamishness, you'll realise that bum is best.

Good luck, and reach out for support if and when you need it.

Sophie Martin @the.infertile.midwife

How counselling can help

Something I'm always struck by when people seek counselling is how often they arrive with a sense of guilt that they 'should' be able to cope more effectively, and that they don't really warrant a counselling session – and that's exactly how I felt when I arrived at my first counselling session, too!

Probably the most important thing for anyone in this situation to understand is that everyone finds infertility and fertility treatments difficult, and that they are very much deserving of additional support at this time.

When can counselling help?

You should be able to access counselling whenever you need it, whether that's before, during or after your treatment. Speak to your clinic early on about the counselling support on offer and how to access it. A readily accessible, highly regarded counselling service is a good indicator of a patient-friendly clinic.

Sometimes people feel guilty about needing counselling or

worried about what it will entail. But it really is your time to use exactly as you'd like without any pressure from anything or anyone else.

Here are just some of the ways that counselling can help during this time:

- You can offload all the toxic emotions you've been carrying. All those feelings that we try so hard to censor when we're with everyone else: the anger, the bitterness, the desperation, the envy, the grief, the guilt and the shame – they can all be shared uncensored with a fertility counsellor.

- You can talk freely in the knowledge that they won't be judging you because they'll understand that these feelings are a normal response to fertility treatments. Rest assured, they will have supported many other women and men who've felt in a similar way to you.

- You can safely confront your fears. The two-week wait is a time of intense highs and lows – and also sleepless nights, where you can't get anxious thoughts out of your mind about what will happen if the cycle hasn't worked. A counsellor won't offer you platitudes but will support you while you explore what lies beneath the fear, enabling you to identify what matters to you and what you need to feel content with your life.

- You can get in touch with your hope. This may sound like a tall order, but often when we've been allowed to release and accept our fears and difficult emotions, our underlying strength starts to emerge – a part of us that can be very helpful to tap into during IVF treatment, and particularly the two-week wait.

- You can explore ways to manage the difficult relationships in your life and nurture the ones that give you strength – all in a way that uniquely suits you and where you are in your life right now.

- You can take back some control. Fertility treatments are overwhelming and most people struggle with so much being out of their hands. Counselling can help you to make peace with the parts of this process that will always fall to chance, and to identify the choices that are still yours to make.

- You can just be you. Most important of all, you can take a break from needing to fit into the role of 'employee', 'partner', 'friend,' and be free to be yourself – whatever that looks like for you at the time of your counselling session. There are no expectations on you for that hour, which can come as a welcome relief during IVF and other fertility treatments.

Rachel Cathan @rachelcathancounselling

When IVF doesn't work...

The bit that no one talks about. We push it to the back of our minds. We try to 'stay positive' and 'hope for the best'. We cling onto our clinic's success rates with every ounce of our being. We try not to think about it not working. But for some, including us, that has become our reality.

Our story began when we discovered we were infertile and needed IVF to conceive. The individual success rate we were given was around thirty per cent. Although we knew deep down that meant a seventy per cent chance of it not working, we tried to stay positive. Where there is life there is hope, as the saying goes, but where there is hope can also be so much pain.

After four years of TTC, we began our first round of IVF on the NHS in January 2018, with a sense of excitement, intrigue and nervousness. The process itself wasn't easy and took almost three months, resulting in just one embryo to transfer on day three. All our hopes were placed on the survival of our little fighter and we thought that maybe, just maybe, it could work.

After the torture of the two-week wait, we were devastated to see just one line on the pregnancy test. I'd seen a lone magpie the day before and knew it was over. There was no fallback, there were no frozen embryos, there was no 'try again' next month. The vast amount of work that had gone into producing our one little embryo would have to be repeated all over again.

The grief we felt was immense as if someone had died, and at first, I couldn't work out why I was feeling so traumatized until I realised I was grieving the loss of a life – an imaginary life, but still a life – the life of our child in our minds. As soon as you imagine what your baby looks like, what it would be like to stroke their hair as they go to sleep, hold them in your arms, hear them cry, wipe their tears, take them to the school gates, picture their first football match, and visualise them grown up … that's when you become a mother. The realisation of that dream not materialising is a huge emotional loss.

We booked a holiday to Turkey in June, just the two of us, to grieve our loss and to rest and prepare for round two. After a relaxing beach holiday, we felt ready to try again and approached round two differently. We knew how devastating the outcome would be if it was negative – we'd been through the tears, the heartbreak and the sleepless nights, so we were less naïve, or so we thought. We protected our feelings by telling ourselves this time that it wouldn't work, but underneath, there was a strong sense of hope.

Our second and last round began in July 2018 with a new protocol of drugs and much trepidation. We produced one more egg than last time so we were hopeful for more embryos, but by day two we were left with just two to transfer, and as advised by our consultant we transferred them both that day. We were hopeful again, knowing we had two chances this time and even entertained the possibility of twins! Our perfect family.

However, two weeks later we discovered another soul-destroying negative. Strangely enough, a lone magpie had appeared in our garden again before OTD (test day), and in my heart I knew. Despite our experience of the grief and despair of our first round, it hit us even harder this time, especially me.

My previous chronic health problems and mental health issues returned, resulting in ten months of sick leave. The effects of the hormones, stress and grief on my body caused a massive relapse. I was numb, lost in the fog of grief. I couldn't see past it; I didn't want to try. I no longer knew who I was, what I wanted or how to fix things. I no longer wanted to be here. I had tried a new antidepressant that was safer in pregnancy, but unfortunately, it had the negative effect of enhancing my already suicidal thoughts and incited a desire to self-harm. I was afraid; afraid of myself and what I might do. Eventually, I was put back onto an antidepressant and several medications for my chronic illnesses that aren't compatible with TTC. It came to the point where it was a matter of life or death. Our only option was to stop IVF so I could continue with the medication. That was and still is our only option. We realised the sanctity of my own life and mental health; I simply couldn't go through it again; my husband and family couldn't see me going through it again. I was at such a low point that I'd completely lost who I was as a person – all my confidence, desire, motivation, happiness and lust for life.

It meant making a sacrifice: giving up the dream of motherhood. I started with small steps and built up until I was able to leave the house again. I began counselling to try and fight my way through the fog of grief, depression, anxiety and the fear of how we'd live our lives without children. I visited a local charity called 'Time Norfolk' who specialise in baby loss, infertility and childlessness.

When I began my counselling sessions I was stuck. I talked about loss and grief all the time and couldn't see a future without children or contemplate moving forward with my life. I honestly felt like life would never be the same again. My counsellor allowed me time to talk; she acknowledged and validated my feelings, but she didn't try to fix them. Over the weeks, she gently asked me to think about the future and what a life without children might look like. I see now that she was challenging me to think about things differently.

My breakthrough moment was the realisation that my past bouts of depression all stemmed from a loss, but not just that, a loss where I had no control of the situation – and IVF was certainly that! I realised how much I'd been through and how that journey shaped the person I am today, and how acceptance and regaining control are key to my recovery. I realised my own strength, that I am 'enough' as I am, that I am 'worthy', and that maybe, just maybe, I could be happy again.

On reflection, it's clear just how much of myself I'd lost to IVF, and if there's one thing to learn from my story, then it's to keep a tight grip on yourself and the things you enjoyed before TTC. Remember to look for joy amongst the cloudiest of skies. Infertility will always be with me; there are reminders everywhere – lone magpies for one! However, two years on from our first round of IVF, I can appreciate the difficult journey we've been on, but also look towards the future and smile.

Emma Manser @finding_my_rainbow

That embryo can be a beautiful healthy child

Hi, my name is Aysha. I'm the mother of a four-year-old boy, a two-year-old girl, and a five-day-old blastocyst that's been in suspended animation for the last six years in a lab, kept at -196 degrees Celsius. No, I'm not a character in some B grade science fiction novel! This is the reality I find myself in as a result of a round of IVF. The IVF was unsuccessful in the end; we had four useable blastocysts, three were implanted with no success, and I had my two children naturally in the end, so we now have one leftover embryo in storage.

Before having IVF, we briefly discussed the possibility of having leftover embryos but it felt like that would be the ultimate best-case scenario, to already have our desired family and still have enough fertilized embryos left over. It was something a little farfetched and too distant in the future to worry about at the time. We didn't dare consider that we'd be so fortunate. After three and a half years of struggling with infertility and being worn down with disappointment and sorrow, our only hope was to have one healthy baby and anything else would be the cherry on our already fabulous cake.

At the time, an embryo was just a microscopic ball of cells. You had to view it that way to protect yourself from the possibility that it might not "take" so you weren't too disappointed. I was told that the chance of IVF success was low anyway as I was approaching forty. I hadn't yet gone through the experience of seeing what a tiny ball of cells can become – a heartbeat at six weeks and then seeing that precious and wondrous embryo develop eyes, a nose, arms and legs, with monthly appointments at the Obstetricians via the black and white haze of an ultrasound. I hadn't yet seen that ball of cells get big enough to smile for the first time or experienced the overwhelming, unconditional love when you finally see that tiny squished up face – and that your love for them continues to grow every day of their lives.

Having two children so close together has been an incredible dream come true, but it's also been a struggle – a beautiful one which I'll never take for granted, in the same way that all mothers who've experienced infertility will never do – but it's a struggle nevertheless. I chose to stay at home and be a full-time mother and it's been difficult without the balance of career and family. I'm not sure I'd have the level of patience and enthusiasm at forty-five to be able to deal with a baby as well as two other young children.

To be brutally honest, I don't want my life to be any more of a struggle than it already is, and I've finally realized how to turn my passion into a career, and that's what I want to focus on for now. I wouldn't consider having a third child at all if it wasn't for this situation. Whenever someone asks me if we're having more children, I get a sense of dread at the thought of it, which is ironic after all those years of longing to be pregnant. So why am I finding it so hard to consider "defrosting" it? Is it because it was so hard-won? I know it's because I see the potential … that this blastocyte can be a beautiful, healthy child that laughs and talks with an adorable lisp like my daughter, or has big green eyes like my son. I see it as a sibling, a playmate for my children, and I wonder what he or she will look like and what personality they'd have? I feel protective of this cluster of cells and that I need to do the right thing by it. I'm it's mother after all and I'm a good mother. I just can't bring myself to let it go. The thought of it makes me so emotional on a deep level.

Donation is out of the question for me, and my clinic doesn't offer it anyway. There's no way I could have my child raised by another family. I'd always be tormented, thinking about my child, wondering if it's loved and happy.

The final option is putting it back, the ultimate roll of the dice, and I'm not much of a gambler. Yes, there's a good chance it might not take and my dilemma would be resolved, but what if it did? Life has a funny way of working sometimes and I'm not ready to take that gamble right now. Although it's been a beautiful struggle, we're a happy little foursome and life is getting easier now that our youngest is almost out of nappies. I'm not willing to rock the boat and throw us back into the disruption of a newborn. Having said all that, I'm open to life's possibilities, and even though I feel this way now, I may not in three months' time.

Aysha O'Connor www.fertilitywithaysha.com

The loss of a cancelled cycle

It took months to feel better after our first IVF cycle had resulted in only one embryo and an early miscarriage. I was broken. Then slowly over time, I managed to pick up the pieces, pull myself back together, and feel stronger emotionally. It helped that we were focused on our next cycle and hopeful that another round would give us a different outcome, or at least more answers.

The day before our first scan, I was anxious about how many follicles we'd have. Would it be more or less than last time? What impact would this have on the success of the cycle? My mind was swimming in unanswered questions, but hopefully, the scan would give us an idea of how things were going. Having been diagnosed with premature ovarian failure earlier that year, I was both managing my expectations but also trying to be hopeful that we'd collect a similar number of eggs as last time.

As the ultrasound technician scanned the first ovary she announced: "Three follicles on the right," and I could feel a tinge of disappointment as I thought back to how many we'd had at this point during our previous cycle, but I was hopeful that the left might have more. As she moved over to the other side I heard: "The left ovary is a bit quieter" followed by, "only one small follicle on that side". My heart sank. This was half as many follicles as we'd had last time at this stage. I knew all too well the harsh reality that not every follicle yields an egg, not every egg collected results in an embryo, not every embryo transferred results in a pregnancy, and not every pregnancy ends with a baby.

I felt our chances slipping through my fingers as I calculated the odds stacked against us. The measurements of each follicle followed, indicating that only one or two were likely to produce eggs. If anything was said to me after this point, I don't remember a single word. My mind was consumed with panic and fear, and all I wanted to do was leave as quickly as I could before anybody saw me cry. I gathered my things and left the clinic, holding back tears as I processed what was happening. I broke down in the doorway of a nearby building and phoned my husband who consoled me as best he could, while strangers walked by staring.

The clinic asked me to return two days later for a further scan, the time in between remaining a painful period of uncertainty and worry. Would we even collect any eggs? Would the cycle be cancelled? Why was this happening to us? We'd put so much time, money, and energy into this cycle already, and now we were facing the prospect that it might not even go ahead. I desperately wanted to know what was going to happen but was also terrified of what the outcome might be.

Two days later the second scan confirmed that at most we'd collect only one egg and the decision was made to cancel the cycle. I felt utterly devastated and drained, both emotionally and physically by the days of not knowing, and now the painful decision to cancel. This was mixed with a strange sense of relief that the uncertainty was over, that however terrible the outcome was, we had a decision and at least knew what was happening.

There was an added grief that this would likely be our last cycle of IVF with my eggs. We knew from everything that happened in the first cycle that our chances of success were low, and hoped the second cycle would give us some much-needed answers to help us move on if it wasn't successful. Financially it wasn't an option for us to continue IVF. Now we were facing the reality that we weren't even able to try this time around and it was completely crushing.

For weeks I buried my grief, choosing to focus on anything I could to keep my mind busy. It took a long time for me to process everything that happened during our cancelled cycle. What surprised me most was that in many ways the cancellation of this cycle hurt just as much as the miscarriage we suffered at the end of our first cycle. The loss of the pregnancy and the loss of this opportunity were both painful in their own way, but they were both losses.

Amelia @infertilebruises

The importance of your mental health and emotional wellbeing

You've decided to go down the path of IVF, maybe not for the first time. You've secured the best clinic for you and you're good to go. Or are you? Something that baffles me is how little attention is given to the emotional impact of IVF, and yet it's vital to your wellbeing and your potential IVF success.

It's crucial to ensure you're emotionally prepared before your IVF treatment commences. This lays down a strong foundation both mentally and physically. Research has shown that including a mind/body connection to your IVF preparation has the potential to double IVF success rates.*

*These studies are small and should be seen as something to be explored rather than proof.

So here are my four key essentials to ensure you're taking care of your emotional wellbeing, in turn enhancing your chances of IVF success.

1. SUCCESS THINKING

Many going through IVF are afraid to get their hopes up because they fear it will hurt too much if their treatment is unsuccessful. Unfortunately, this has the potential to send conflicting messages to your body about whether it's useful to become pregnant. I'm sure you're wondering why that is, so let me explain.

When we're anxious and afraid, we move into an emergency state where the ancient 'feeling' part of our brain perceives physical danger. If a woman were in real physical danger, the last thing she'd need for survival would be pregnancy, hence the conflicting messages being passed through to her body.

I'm sure you're now asking yourself how to avoid this because IVF treatment itself can be incredibly stressful, and it can be hard not to fear failure, can't it? The answer is knowing you can 'handle it' if you don't get the result you hoped for. Let me prove to you that you can 'handle it'.

I'm pretty sure you've had emotional pain in your life before, haven't you? Difficult situations that you thought you may never get over. In challenging times, we have no choice but to get on and 'handle it,' and so we do.

Preparing for failure doesn't stop the pain

Inevitably you're going to hurt if your IVF treatment isn't successful. Therefore, instead of avoiding feeling hopeful, it's better to acknowledge that there is HOPE and you will become pregnant. At the same time, acknowledge that if it doesn't happen, you'll work through the pain in the same way you've worked through other emotional pain you've experienced. In other words, you will handle it.

My suggestion is to write down the following statement and place it somewhere visible for you to see every day:

"Whilst I'm going through IVF, I acknowledge there is HOPE that I will become pregnant. If that doesn't happen, I know I can handle it because I've handled everything life has thrown at me to date."

2. SUCCESS STEPS

Going through IVF can be overwhelming, can't it? There is, after all, so much to do:

- Injections that you have to work around your daily life.

- Appointments that are hard to explain away, especially if you're having to take time off work, or cancel meet-ups at short notice when no one knows that you're going through IVF.

- Procedures that can feel scary and emotional, either because they're the first time you're having them or because you've done it way too many times before.

- Waiting when time seems to standstill.

Whenever we feel overwhelmed, the best thing we can do for ourselves is to make a plan. When working with my fertility clients, we lay out what I call 'Success Steps', to plan out how they're going to handle all these things. It's worth you working through the logistics so you feel in control.

Depending on where you are on your journey, you may not know your future plans, which is fine. Clarify what you do know and add to your Success Steps as you discover more.

3. SELF-CARE STRATEGY

Having a daily self-care strategy is a useful way to help relax both your body and mind. I teach my clients three ways to do this.

- Daily Dump – at least once a day spend time writing down any negative thoughts. It's as simple as dumping everything that comes up – a flow of moans if you like. This is NOT journaling, which is more about focusing on what you do want. Think of it as dumping all of the toxic energies in your head.

- Daily Dancing – sticking on a great tune and having a boogie is a great way to change your mental state and lift your mood.

- Daily Downtime – at least once a day, take half an hour to listen to something relaxing, allowing yourself to let go and unwind.

4. SIXTH SENSE

This may sound a bit woo-woo, but it's a useful decision-making tool. What I'm talking about is using your gut instincts to make the right choices. Our intuition always wants to guide us, even if the noise of our worries might drown them out. Fortunately, you can train yourself to listen to your sixth sense.

Start by taking a nice relaxing breath in, then ask yourself what your next best steps are. As you breathe out, notice what comes in first: 'YES' or 'NO'. I want you to be mindful, though, that as soon as you get that first answer, the analytical part of your brain will kick in and start questioning. That's why breathing is useful because it quietens the mind so you can hear that first answer. All you have to do is LISTEN.

This can be useful if you haven't yet decided on the elements of your treatment. If you're in the early stages of this process it could be about what clinic to attend, a particular protocol, and even what holistic support you may want to use, such as working with a Fertility Coach, having Acupuncture, Reflexology, or seeing a Nutritionist, etc.

SUMMARY

In conclusion, don't underestimate the importance of your emotional wellbeing, and the mind/body connection toward your IVF treatment and its potential success. Implementing four simple elements before commencing IVF has the potential to greatly increase your chances of success, and prevent your treatment from affecting your mental health.

Here's a reminder of what they are:

1. Success Thinking – ensure that you're sending the right messages to your body about getting pregnant.

2. Success Steps – to avoid feeling overwhelmed.

3. Self-Care Strategy – ensure that you're physically and emotionally calm throughout your treatment.

4. Sixth Sense – tap into your gut instincts to ensure you make all the right decisions for you.

I hope you've found learning about my four key essentials interesting, and that they prove useful during your IVF treatment and your ongoing fertility journey.

Dany Griffiths @freedomfertilityformula

Negative feelings

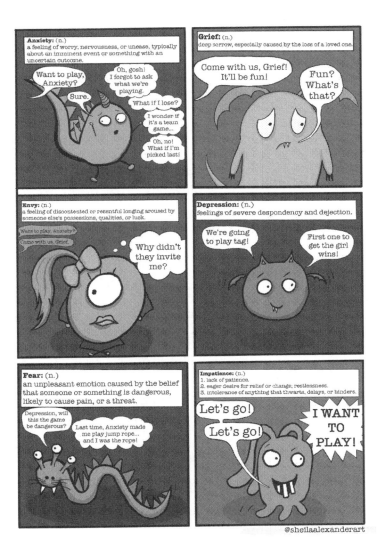

@sheilaalexanderart

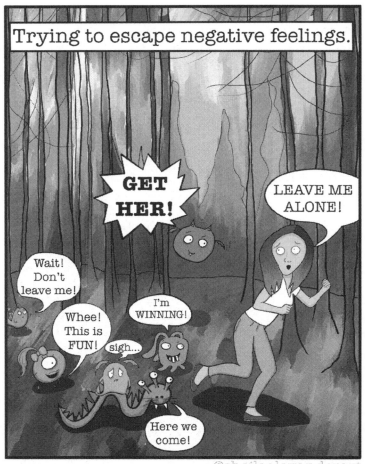

The financial costs of IVF in the UK

Like most countries, fertility clinics are free to set their own costs just like any other private healthcare provider. This means that the same treatment could be two or even three times more expensive depending on which clinic you choose. It's strongly recommended that you shop around before committing to a clinic and consider a wide range of factors, not just the financial, when making your final decision. A lot of clinics hold free open evenings so you can go along, meet the team and ask questions.

Some clinics may quote a cost that's for the treatment only, such as IVF or ICSI, and not fertility drugs, (which can be very expensive), freezing leftover embryos or other administration costs. Others may quote for everything and therefore seem more expensive at first glance. Drugs don't have to be ordered from your clinic, there are alternative pharmacy companies that supply the same drugs cheaper. Therefore, ensure you're comparing like with like.

The HFEA (Human Fertilisation & Embryology Authority) are a Government regulator and they charge the fertility clinics for each IVF and IUI cycle they perform which covers the regulation costs. Despite some clinics listing this on their bill, the HFEA aren't charging you.

Over and above the costs for a standard IVF or ICSI cycle are the costs of what are called 'add-ons'. Some clinics include them in the cost of a cycle, whereas others charge separately, and they can be expensive. The HFEA advises that there is no conclusive evidence that some of the commonly offered add-ons increase the chance of pregnancy, so it's your choice if you want to pay for them, but as long as you understand the evidence, (which is on their website), you'll be able to make an informed decision.

The following costs are approximate and are just to give you a very rough idea:

Initial fertility clinic consultation: £265

One Clomid cycle: £400

IUI cycle – scans, blood tests, sperm preparation, procedure: £1,430.00

Drugs from the clinic for an IUI cycle: £320 - £565

IVF cycle – scans, blood tests, egg collection and day 3 transfer, pregnancy scan, follow-up consultation, x1 counselling session: £4,030

IVF cycle - scans, blood tests, egg collection and day 5 transfer, pregnancy scan, follow-up consultation, x1 counselling session: £4,600

Medications from the clinic for an IVF cycle: £900 - £2,250

ICSI – extra to IVF: £1,250

PGD Testing for five embryos: from £2,300 - £4,500

Frozen Embryo Transfer – scans, blood tests, transfer, pregnancy scan, follow up consultation, x1 counselling session: £1,900

Embryo freezing and one - year storage: £900

Dietary supplements (approx.) per cycle: £300

Approximate cost of three, day five, IVF cycles, medications and three years of embryo freezing is £23,595.00

It isn't unusual for the first IVF cycle not to work; often someone has to complete at least three cycles before they get a positive pregnancy test. Even though they may get this far, it isn't definite that they'll get to nine months and bring their baby home. For some, their cycles will run into double figures and they may still not take a baby home.

From the beginning of an IVF cycle to embryo transfer, a lot of women choose alternative therapies to support the process, such as acupuncture, reflexology, hypnotherapy and coaching. Everyone having fertility treatments are advised to have counselling, and should be offered it through their clinic - some include one session in their treatment price. If you have more sessions this will be an additional cost and varies from each practitioner. Some people will receive fertility treatment for free on the NHS, but it varies as to where you live and eligibility is difficult.

Whatever country you live in, if you find yourself heading down the IVF route, the cost is more than you expect, and many cannot afford to even do one cycle. A lot of people take out a bank loan or ask parents or relatives for financial help. And remember, there's no guarantee that you will have a baby.

Sheila @fertilitybooks

The financial costs of IVF in the U.S

There are two costs where IVF are concerned: the emotional and the financial. They're usually connected for obvious reasons. I've detailed below the average cost in the U.S of fertility care today, over a three-year journey.

I've found that most of my US clients have insurance, but there's no fertility cover included. This means that the insurance will often cover blood work, hormone and thyroid tests, sperm analysis, and sometimes ultrasounds, depending on the underlying factor causing infertility and how 'creative' the clinic gets with billing. My hysteroscopy, laparoscopies with ablation, and HSG (hysterosalpingogram) were covered by my insurance.

The following is an example of the average costs over three years:

Initial Consult: $350

4 cycles timed intercourse with the drug Clomid: $200

2 IUI's, necessary ultrasounds, meds Letrazole and trigger shot: $2,100

2 IUI's, necessary ultrasounds with injectable meds and trigger shot: $3,500

Dietary supplements: $1,000

12 months counselling: $720

IVF, necessary ultrasounds, "freeze all": $14,000

IVF medications: $4,000

PGD testing: $5,000

Embryo freezing and one-year storage: $1,000

2 Frozen embryo transfers: $10,000

Total Cost: $41,870

OK, I know it's expensive. I can't, unfortunately, do much about the price, but I can provide you with some tips to make this more manageable.

Top three tips:

1) Ask the right cost questions

The very first question to ask is if the fertility clinic consultation is free. If it's not, will they put the cost of it as a credit towards future services?

Next, make sure the clinic is upfront about their pricing. Although some variables are impossible to predict – medication for example – they should have a price sheet and be able to give you a range of what to expect. If a clinic seems hesitant to share, run in the other direction.

I'd also ask how they bill the insurance company for underlying conditions. Even if you don't have fertility coverage benefits, treatment of conditions contributing to/causing infertility might be covered. For instance, because of my endometriosis, all of my ultrasounds for monitoring were covered. We also had benefits for blood draws and semen analysis because of my 'creative' billing.

A question you'll need to ask is: "How can I lower my costs?" For example, does the clinic have a donated med program? Do they have information on manufacturer discount programs? Are they participating in any upcoming clinical trials?

2) Make more money

Start charging for consulting in your area of expertise. Sell your stuff online via FB Marketplace, Mercari, or eBay. Sell your stuff in person at a consignment shop or yard sale. Ask your boss for a raise if you haven't had one yet. If you're in the U.S. check out missingmoney.com to see if your state owes you any cash. There are a ton of ways to make moolah quickly – but the money in hand is only a small part of the real benefits. The magic happens when you shift your momentum. When you take back control and prove to yourself that you CAN do this and that you're dedicated to making it happen one step at a time.

3) Have a visual savings tool

You can make your own or print mine off for free here: DevonBaeza.com/15crazyways – which work on a lot of different levels psychologically.

- Stating your goals in writing makes it more of a reality

- Coloring in the pyramid with each dollar you save gives your brain a quick 'win'. The process reprograms the reward center in your brain to choose saving money over the instant gratification of a small purchase

- Placing it somewhere you can see it multiple times a day

reinforces what matters most and removes competing priorities

- Being clear about the EXACT amount of money you want and a deadline date to receive it helps manifest what you most desire. It's like putting in an order to the universe! I love seeing what crazy fun things happen for clients when they start focusing on manifesting.

I know it's difficult when you're in the middle of treatment, overwhelmed, and stressed to the max financially. I promise it won't always be this hard. Hang in there! Don't let money stop you from enjoying motherhood.

Devon Baeza @the_fertility_finance_coach

For seventy per cent of people, IVF doesn't work

My husband and I have been trying for seven years and still no baby, and struggling to have a family has changed me immeasurably. It's negatively impacted my mental, emotional and financial health, put huge pressure on my relationship with my husband, and at times, I have sunk so low, I've wanted to lay down and die.

IVF will work for thirty per cent of women and that figure reduces after the age of thirty-five. Thirty per cent – did you know that figure? Because we didn't. I was thirty-seven when we started trying for a family. That means for seventy per cent of people, IVF won't work. Why doesn't anyone tell you that? Why doesn't the GP when you tell them you've been trying for a year and nothing is happening? Why doesn't the gynaecologist say when you get your tubes checked or the fertility nurse when you're considering options and eligibility? Once you've moved on from the NHS to private, no-one is going to tell you because then you're in a huge money-making business; a bottomless black hole of hopes and dreams and tens of thousands of pounds.

Trying to conceive is an emotionally draining process from the first time you research all the possible clinics, visit them, and decide on the one where the stats are good, and you can drive to easily and park. I didn't want to use public transport just in case I received bad news at an appointment; going home by car was much more preferable. Multiple people recommended the clinic we chose, and the staff were friendly and empathic all the way through to the test date of every cycle.

The first time you're shown the video on how to administer the injections, it's exciting ... there's hope, although there's bruising and swelling, slightly improved by icing your stomach before an injection. My husband gave them to me every day so that he was part of our journey; from one brand of meds for the first cycle, to the brand changing and adding in Heparin for our last protocol, the fourth or fifth time ... I lose track. Throughout, your body and mind are on a complete rollercoaster, your hormones all over the place. One day you're OK, the next you're crying for no reason. Your tummy is itchy, bruised and swollen, and all the time you're trying to maintain a job and stay hopeful for the baby, the family you're desperately trying to create.

The scans went well, revealing my womb lining was thickening as it should, getting ready for egg collection. I then waited patiently for the phone call the next day. With our first IVF cycle, the embryos weren't great – we only got a few good ones and they didn't develop as hoped, so we had one put back in on day 2 – it could work, we told ourselves. We had hope.

Writing this so many years later from when we first started investigations and treatment, you forget the intricate details, the names of the drugs, the days when things happened. You just remember how it all made you feel: drained, your confidence crushed with deep sadness, frustration and anger. I made a box of everything to do with our fertility journey. It's in a cupboard put away: a box of pain and upset. IVF is a peculiar experience; you're aware of so much more than when you conceive naturally. Day one of the life of a potential baby, days when you're classed as pregnant until proven otherwise (i.e. test day), that dreaded two-week wait when you work out the approximate date when your baby will be due. You become an expert, you scrutinise the minutiae, you overanalyse everything, and the more you do this, the more emotional you become.

We've seen specialist after specialist, consultants, experts at a variety of fertility clinics, Harley Street offices, a nutritionist, acupuncturist, reflexologist, went through years of fertility counselling and attended groups, my husband always being the only male. All of these people keeping our hopes alive and none of them, I feel, stating the facts or being honest about our situation. I've had operations, invasive investigations and blood tests. In the beginning, some were on the NHS, some were classed as 'gynaecological' and were paid for by our private health insurance, but most cost us thousands for all the treatment, drugs and scans.

Through this journey, we found out the multitude of things that can affect conceiving and incubation of a potential baby, and when these things fail at an early stage, as they have for us, you go through a grieving process for something that, if you conceived naturally, you'd be completely oblivious about.

It's been a gruelling process; we've decided not to continue, although with time and a year's bereavement counselling, we've decided to use our two frozen embryos this year (we created donor embryos due to recommendations around my age). There's some glimmer of hope. If it works or doesn't work, 2020 must be my year of acceptance. The grief and pain have dominated my life so significantly, I must find joy in other ways.

Lauren Juggler Crook

Focusing on what you can control

When my husband and I embarked on the journey of IVF, I understood the importance of my role in this process. I knew there was a lot I could control. Often, I see women giving their power away, assuming their doctors and/or clinics hold all the solutions. To an extent, yes, they play a huge role in using modern medicine through advanced assisted reproductive technology, (ART), however, you also hold the key. I want to spread the message that you have a lot more control in this process than you realize. I'm here to inspire you to consider the impact of your mindset, the energy you bring to this process, and your daily practices of self-care. They matter more than you know.

The IVF rollercoaster ride is one of the most transformative experiences you will ever go on. What drives me is helping women, like you, see their fertility journey as one of hope and possibility. It can be joyful, and it can also be magical, however, we're not led to believe it can be this way. Learning that we had one healthy embryo after two egg retrievals and PGS (pre-implantation genetic screening) testing was all I needed to keep hope alive. Through many setbacks – having three unexpected surgeries including removal of uterine polyps, scar tissue removal, and removal of uterine fibroids, my husband and I remained faithful that our little one was there waiting for us.

What I knew I could control were my thoughts – mindset is so crucial. I developed strong self-awareness to recognize that the energy I carried with me in my regular monitoring appointments and how I felt while taking my medications mattered. My husband was extremely supportive throughout our whole journey, but I knew a lot of it was on me. My body was the one receiving and reacting to the hormones and I was also the one undergoing all the procedures. I chose to give myself my own shots, which was liberating, and I took control by also staying on top of all my scheduled appointments.

Practicing self-care was essential throughout the entire process and especially in recovery from all my surgeries. The waiting periods were often long, yet, I understood the importance of tending to my mental, spiritual and emotional wellbeing. I believe the emotional pain is truly one of the hardest parts of this process, but there is a way through without losing yourself.

Some ideas on how I took control of my IVF pathway:

- regular journaling
- focusing on mantras to help keep me in a positive frame of mind
- holistic practices such as acupuncture and reiki
- having a strong support network and sisterhood.

One of the keys to finding peace within this process is to surrender to what you can't control while focusing on what you can control. It's essential to 'let go' of trying to control too much. Remember, YOU are responsible for the thoughts you are thinking. YOU are responsible for the energy you bring to this process. YOU can control how you react to the setbacks that happen. And it's YOU that needs to make self-care a priority.

My background as an occupational therapist for the past twenty years helped me immensely in utilizing a holistic approach in my fertility journey. As a mother to our two-year-old, our one healthy embryo, I'm passionate about supporting others on this path. If you're feeling hopeless and overwhelmed, I highly suggest talking with others who've been on this journey and have knowledge to share. I'm here for you!

Lisa White @IVF.manifesting.a.miracle

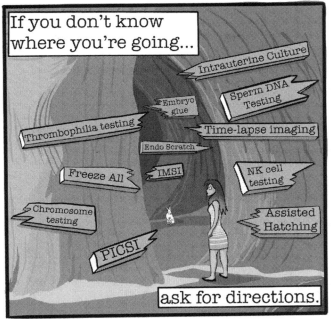

If you don't know where you're going... ask for directions.

Intrauterine Culture · Sperm DNA Testing · Embryo glue · Thrombophilia testing · Time-lapse imaging · Endo Scratch · IMSI · NK cell testing · Freeze All · Chromosome testing · Assisted Hatching · PICSI

@sheilaalexanderart

Secondary infertility and IVF

Dear Friend,

Most people look at me and see two beautiful, healthy twin girls and a loving husband. And while all that's true, what they don't see is what's been going on every day for the past two and a half years.

Let's rewind to nine years ago when we were trying to have a child. I wasn't having periods naturally, and still don't, so I resorted to fertility treatments. As a twenty-seven-year-old, this was challenging. But we did it! We went to the fertility center and figured out a plan. Maybe it's because we were so young, hopeful and healthy, but we were fortunate to conceive twins via IUI (intrauterine insemination), on the first try. So, while we dealt with medications and the stress of infertility, we were the lucky ones for whom treatment worked successfully.

Fast forward to today: two and a half years of trying to conceive baby #3. While we knew we'd have to go through treatments again, we never imagined still being here. Between the daily appointments, the financial burden, time away from my children and the emotional roller coaster of what is IVF, this has truly taken its toll on me and my family. Needless to say, I'm in a constant state of GUILT.

You see, it's different than going through infertility treatments when you don't have any children. For starters, yes, it IS easier because I DO have two amazing daughters who I'm so thankful for. But, therein lies the guilt. Every single day I choose to move forward with treatments and take time away from my daughters. I force myself to put on a brave face, no matter what's going on. I hide in my room and cry, take my shots and talk to the doctor from my closet so they don't hear or see me. I often have to bring my daughters with me to appointments, and it scares them to know mommy is at the doctor's again. So, you see, it's different. It's not just me and my future baby I have to think about, it's me and my current family that I have to prioritize. For us, IVF comes second, and that's a challenge.

Sadly, people are also much less compassionate when it comes to my situation. "Well at least you already have two daughters," some say. My heart drops to my stomach and all I can do is nod and answer, "I know." But I want to scream and say: "One has nothing to do with the other! Don't you know how much stuff you're dumping on me?" But of course, I never say that because guilt takes over. It's a constant battle that goes on in my head, and it's a very lonely one.

I'm also at the point in my life where so many of my friends are having their second, third or fourth babies, and while I'm happy for them, it's also hard to be around them. I've distanced myself from certain people and become very close to others who truly are supportive. I suppose that's a good thing, but baby showers, holidays and baby announcements make me sad.

And finally, there's the financial stress. How can I put my family through this and diminish what we've worked so hard for, for something that doesn't exist, yet? MORE GUILT. IVF is expensive and every time we sign the dotted line for a new cycle, a scan, an MRI exam or a test, I feel as though I'm sacrificing things my family need.

Secondary infertility is different. It's not me wanting to be a mom, because, thankfully, I already am a mom. It's me wanting to expand my family. It comes with a stigma because I should be happy and grateful for what I've got. And there isn't a single day that I don't thank my lucky stars for the life I have. But yearning for another child and going through so many losses is something society doesn't seem to understand.

And yet, here I am, still pushing on, because, after a lot of therapy, I know this is my story. I know, I deserve this child, and I know my family understands. And one day, I'll know that all of this was worth the fight, the tears, the stress and the arguments. This new baby will be part of our family and we'll have a strong bond because of this journey ... a bond that most families aren't lucky enough to enjoy. Silver lining.

Erin Bulcao @mybeautifulblunder

The benefits of an IVF planner

I have a membership in the '1 in 8' Infertility Club. After trying to conceive the 'natural way' for almost two years and finding out that the only way to motherhood in my case was IVF (in vitro fertilization), it was really hard and devastating.

My first four cycles were extremely stressful and difficult. The first one obviously because I didn't know what to expect. The second cycle was cancelled due to an error the clinic made – they switched my meds chart with another patient and told me the wrong dose to inject, so I got OHSS (Ovarian hyperstimulation syndrome) which is potentially life-threatening. My third cycle ended with the stillbirth of my beautiful baby girl, Isabelle, at thirty-nine weeks. In desperation, I did my fourth cycle almost immediately after losing Isabelle and even though I got a BPF (big fat positive pregnancy result), I miscarried at seven weeks. I was devastated again, but I believe it was down to being a mess emotionally, physically and mentally.

Yes. Infertility sucks! But all our struggles taught me and my hubby a lot. Not only that, but it also inspired me to open up about my journey to motherhood and coach others walking the same path. It also encouraged me to write my book *The IVF Planner, a personal journal to organize your journey through in-vitro fertilization (IVF) with love and positivity,* a must-have for anyone going through IVF. I truly recommend you have a planner during this time, because trust me, keeping up with the appointments, how many meds to take and when, and other information will help you, not only with being able to manage the stress, but also, it's a way to write your own story, and one day be able to show your baby how incredible the road was to bring him/her into the world.

I realized that a planner is not only a tool for journaling but also a unique and personal coaching tool. Having a planner helps to take control of the situation you're going through. In my case, it helped me to accept my medical situation, my menstrual cycles, my body, my feelings, as well as my relationship with my hubby. It was like having a coach right when I needed them. So, by being aware that I can't control the waiting time, it was better that I became creative and found other opportunities.

Any fertility treatment, but especially IVF, brings extra stress to not only the woman but also her partner. With IVF comes many emotions, including a sense of being overwhelmed and confused. The fact that I had detailed information about my cycle also helped me communicate easily with my RE, nurses and the clinic. I was able to keep track of my questions and sometimes even find the answers myself as a result of tracking them.

Each of us suffering from infertility issues have different experiences, feelings and emotions during treatment. Each case and each cycle are unique. There's no way to know exactly how the various aspects of the treatment (medical, emotional, psychological, financial and physical), will affect each individual.

Fertility Coaching, especially from someone having experienced it, can help anyone walking the same path, giving them a more constructive approach to IVF and infertility. It can help create positive thought patterns, organize finances better, and allow us to see all the blessings and knowledge available to make this journey a more joyful one.

Women going through IVF and their partners are made of courage and strength. We've been given this mission for a reason … I've learned that from my own experience, and trust me, it's worth it. Always remember that this journey, no matter the end result – negative, positive or cancelled cycles – takes strength and courage, and teaches us to be disciplined, patient and kinder.

Monica Bivas @monicabivas

I just want to be a Mum

Based on the blog 'IVF – the beginning'

It was May 2016 that Dorothea was created, but our journey started long before that.

As an older couple we didn't want to hang around waiting for the 'right time' to try for a baby, so, we decided early in our relationship to come off contraception and let 'nature' run its course. And we waited and waited … but nothing happened.

We decided to use a fertility app and I peed on ovulation sticks as well as continually having sex, but nearly a year later, still nothing.

We visited the GP and had some basic fertility checks, blood tests and a semen analysis. We were referred for fertility treatment in April 2015 after tests revealed male factor infertility; analysis showed a near-normal count but low 'normal forms,' meaning that although natural conception was possible, it was unlikely. Following more bloods and tests ruling out STDs and other infectious diseases, specialist fertility blood tests and ovarian scans, we were ready to go ahead with a funded IVF cycle.

We were referred to a local fertility clinic to begin the process. I was told my AMH (anti-Mullerian hormone) levels were high, indicating a good reserve of eggs, but that this possibly indicated PCOS (polycystic ovary syndrome). Further sperm analysis revealed a range of figures which confused us and didn't seem related to any health or lifestyle changes we'd made. Due to sperm quality, we needed to have ICSI, which is when the selected sperm is injected into the egg.

Our first cycle started in October 2015, a few days after a lovely holiday and my birthday. Despite that relaxing interval, I still felt stressed and had more responsibility at work which increased the pressure I was under. I also hadn't done much research and was trying to 'go with the flow,' but every appointment was met with anxiety and tears, despite my partner trying to relax me.

IVF treatment involves a range of drugs and treatments from self-administered injections to tablets, nasal sprays and vaginal pessaries or rectal suppositories. The box of supplies for a cycle is overwhelming: a huge number of unfamiliar drugs with a scary quantity of needles and syringes! I was fine with the needles and drugs, I'm a nurse, so this part of the process didn't bother me at all. It was the mental pressure – after wanting to be a mum for so many years, I was nervous it wouldn't work and it was hard to relax.

The injections were ongoing to grow the follicles and

mature the eggs. At each appointment, there were thirty to forty follicles – a high number – normally, there'd be ten to twenty follicles. They said I was at risk of OHSS (ovarian hyperstimulation syndrome) and wanted to monitor me closely. They reduced my dose of the stimulation drugs to help lower the risk. I cannot describe the feeling of huge fluid-filled ovaries. It felt weird and uncomfortable. The nurse told me my ovaries were around the size of walnuts but after seven days of stimulating drugs, mine were the size of large oranges! When I walked quickly, I could feel them bouncing inside me and I was told no running or activity due to a risk of torsion – which means twisting.

So, I had a scan and some blood tests on a Friday, and in the clinic, the following Monday, my scan revealed a shock – massive follicles! The nurse was surprised, saying she was unsure how they'd grown so much on a reduced dose. What! I'd not been told to adjust my dose. It turns out they'd left a voicemail to halve my stim dose that I'd never received. I was told to stop the stims and await blood results. A call came later to say that my hormone levels were dangerously high – they were 21,000 and should be less than 17,000. I had to return to the clinic and was given a drug called Cabergoline to counteract the effect and hopefully stop the likelihood of OHSS. I took the drug but was scared, and I still had to return to my nursing job.

I quickly felt unwell, collapsing and vomiting at work. Nick, my partner, had to come and collect me. I had such severe vertigo and sickness that I could only lie flat or crawl. I'd never felt so ill. The clinic said it was a severe allergic reaction to the drug and that I needed to drink three to four litres of water a day.

After two days of severe sickness I had my egg collection; twenty eggs were retrieved from thirty-one follicles. To collect the eggs, they insert a dildo-like implement into your vagina and then poke a needle through your vaginal wall and into each ovary, sucking out the contents of each plump follicle. I was sedated so I didn't recall a thing. Afterwards, there was just period type cramps and blood spotting.

After the great news of twenty eggs, seventeen were mature and yet only seven fertilised. It was demoralising! We'd hoped to get at least fifty per cent. Then we had to wait for a call, hoping that day by day the cells in the embryos would divide normally. The aim is to get them to a five-day embryo, called a blastocyst. On day three, the clinic called. We only had three embryos left in the running, and they weren't brilliant quality. We were advised to come in for the transfer. The risk was that we could wait until day five, and there would be no embryo to transfer. We were gutted.

I remember crying en-route to the hospital. Nick played my 'relaxing IVF app' but it didn't help … I was in pieces. Two embryos were transferred: a 'good' eight-cell embryo and a fragmented ten-cell, meaning the cells inside the embryo are irregular in shape. I remember Nick asking the doctor what we could do to improve our chances … should I rest etc. She replied: 'Either you get pregnant or you don't.'

Then came the dreaded two-week wait, the most awful time, when you question every potential symptom. Do I have sore boobs, any pain, is my period coming? Eleven days later, we got our answer when we returned to the clinic – it hadn't worked! A urine and blood test confirmed it. We went home to cry.

Not only had this cycle not worked, but it was our only funded cycle; our only chance of getting pregnant on the NHS. What millions of couples take for granted, having a family, meant suddenly we had to find thousands of pounds.

Yes, infertility sucks! It affects you mentally, physically and financially. It challenges your relationship, can make you seriously ill, and feel like a total failure! Why can't I do what we're put on this earth for? I just want a baby, a family.

Kelly @ivf.ninja

(Link to the blog: http://motherhoodafterivf.com/2019/05/07/ivf-the-beginning/)

The perfect conception vessel

I was mentally exhausted, my body felt defeated, and I needed to stop … to break the cycle we were in. Unsuccessful IVF attempts month after month meant we needed to press reset.

When you're trying to conceive you can put immense pressure on yourself to create the 'perfect vessel'. You get overwhelmed with far too many opinions, wanted and unwanted, and will try anything and everything: eating foods that are suggested for fertility and avoiding others, doing juice detox's, trying meditation and fertility acupuncture as well as limiting intense exercise … the list goes on. All of this means that you're not doing it for you! As a result, you've created even more stress than you started with, which is the exact opposite of what you want to achieve.

Overall wellness relies on a balanced synergy between your mind, body and emotions. This balance can be disrupted when you're in the 'trying to conceive' cycle. It wasn't until I hit pause on 'trying' that I realised how disconnected I was from myself. It then hit me. I needed to shift my focus towards doing the things that my mind, body and emotions craved, not what I thought I needed, to create the perfect conception vessel.

At this stage, I discovered my love for yoga. It was a beautiful mix of physical strength-building for my body, tranquillity for my mind, and gave me a deeper core connection to what some would call soul. It was my opportunity to step away from the outside world and listen to what was going on internally, and the first chance I'd had to nurture myself in a really long time. I consciously took time to pause, listen, and stop ignoring the voice within that was screaming at me to give my mind and body a rest from trying so hard to conceive.

It was during a yoga class that I learnt the meaning of the beautiful Sanskrit word Santosha, meaning:'To live in complete contentment and acceptance. A deep state of inner peace.' It resonated with me immediately. I was so far from living in a state of Santosha, but I knew immediately that it was this mantra that I needed to live and breathe before I welcomed our next baby. I'd been focusing way too much on what I didn't have in my life – a sibling for my daughter. My tunnel vision was blocking me from finding happiness in the beauty I already had right in front of me. Trying to conceive for such a long time had created a dark cloud and I needed it to vanish.

By slowly shifting my thinking and practising living in a state of Santosha, I began to free myself from the desperation to have another baby. It allowed me to accept whatever circumstances presented: including pleasure, pain, success or failure. It helped me develop a better relationship with myself. I got better at accepting and being happy the way things were in the present moment, rather than making happiness dependent on achieving certain goals or changing aspects of myself.

Hindsight is a beautiful gift and now my greatest teacher. Trying to conceive can put our minds into a deep state of lack, because of the desperation of wanting something that is out of our control.

If you're feeling unhappy, I encourage you to pause for a moment and change your focus. Start by finding contentment in the little things that make you smile from within. Acknowledge what you're already grateful for. Be gentle with yourself and find ways to reconnect with the things that bring you immense joy. It won't take away the emotional and physical pain that arises from IVF or the journey to conceive, but it will help your heart to open for whatever is next on your fertility journey.

Adriana Michael @stateofsantosha

Frozen in hope

When we were trying to fall pregnant with our first child all manner of fears swept through me … what if we can't get pregnant? What will we do then? Would we need someone else's genetic material to help us? And how would that impact on this ideal family we'd dreamt of becoming? How would it feel to have unrelated children? Would it make any difference?

We struggled on with our own eggs and sperm … and got lucky. Our second round of harvested eggs gave us three great embryos. We begged the doctors to let us have two of them put back in me. We had to sign all sorts of multiple birth waivers, but they agreed. The third embryo was frozen.

And hooley dooley we got twins! They were large as life on the screen at our seven-week scan, reminding me of tiny seahorses with their hearts blipping on the screen in green against the black background. I wish I'd remembered my phone so I could record it because by the eleven-week scan there was only one. It was a bittersweet day for us. I truly had to grieve the one we'd just lost. I felt it was necessary, given that I hadn't dealt well with our last miscarriage, and so I could fully appreciate the gift of the remaining baby.

We hadn't found out the sex on purpose as everything else had been so damned medical and planned that we, actually I, wanted a bit of suspense and romance about this one aspect. Would it matter if we had a boy or a girl? We were having a baby! It could have been a puppy for all I cared at that point.

He was born in November of 2012. And we called him Luke – partly because it was the only boys' name we'd agreed on the entire pregnancy, and Luke sounds like 'lucky,' and we felt so lucky to be out the other side, finally holding our baby.

His infancy was wonderful and as he grew, we got those pangs of wondering whether we'd put ourselves through it all again to complete our family with a sibling. Of course, we would, and we were super lucky that when Luke was weaning, we fell pregnant – All On Our Own! We were amazed and a bit miffed – so my body knew how to do it now. What about before? But also, thrilled not to have to go through all the needles, the prodding, the doctors being too involved, again. I can't even tell you how good that felt.

The week before Christmas 2014, we welcomed our second miracle – a girl, we named, Keira. This birth had been hard on me physically, requiring significant surgical repair that I was advised wouldn't withstand another birth.

Then after she was born, we received a letter from our fertility clinic asking us to decide whether to continue storing the embryo we had in their freezer. And it occurred to us that we were a complete family: the two of us and our two kids. Yet, we knew there were many more people out there who weren't. And we couldn't just let our embryo defrost. We'd been through too much to create it. We'd seen how much egg donation had meant to some close family and friends who'd had their own long and winding fertility journey. So, when faced with the decision of what to do with our extra embryo, it was a no-brainer. Our two healthy, happy kids are pretty wonderful and the thought that someone else could experience that same happiness is all we needed to donate our last embryo to help others.

We met with a clinic that specialises in donations and went to meetings to ensure we were completely set on the idea of handing over our genetic material to another family. During those discussions we learned a lot about what it means to be a legal family, and that any resulting child would not technically be related to us – we'd have no rights to meet with them, or legal obligations to them either. But we did provide details to the clinic about us and the kind of people we are, so that if one day the resulting child wanted to learn more about their genetic history, or reach out to meet us, then they could. We will probably never know who received our cluster of cells. It's probably better that we don't, but I sincerely hope it worked out for them.

We chose not to put restrictions on who the clinic could give our embryo to, because love is love. They could be single, a hetero couple, or any other type of family. We trusted that the clinic would make it available to someone in real need, who'd be sure that it was the right thing for both them and the child.

So far, we've chosen not to call the clinic and see if anything came of our donation. I like to believe that we did a good and noble thing, and the result is something separate. It's a bit like Schrodinger's cat experiment – there either is or isn't another child out there made with our recipe, but once I ask the question of the clinic, I can't unknow the result. And if it didn't work out, what then? Guilt for putting someone through another loss? It may be a romantic notion but I choose to believe it worked out, because I'd hate to think that it didn't, having known what it's like to have lost babies too.

For now, I've put the clinic's number in my phone, and one day I might call. But not today. I want to hope, just a little longer.

Sandi Friedlos @sandifriedlos

Waiting for PGS results

There is A LOT of 'waiting' when you're doing fertility treatment; waiting for test results, waiting to start IVF, waiting for egg collection, waiting to find out how your embryos are developing… even waiting in clinic waiting rooms! There is the well-known 'two-week wait' or 2WW, which is when you wait to do a pregnancy test roughly two-weeks after your embryo is transferred, to find out if this cycle has been successful. But there is another, lesser known two-week wait which is equally hard to get through, and this is for PGS* (Preimplantation Genetic Screening) results – your blastocysts have been biopsied to test if they are chromosomally normal, or not - and you are waiting for THOSE results!

The wait itself is similar to the dreaded 2WW and I'd recommend doing pretty much the same things to pass the time and to prepare for transfer – rest, relax, eat, and do only the things you love to do.

So why have PGS? My first ever pregnancy turned out to be ectopic and I underwent surgery to remove my left fallopian tube where the embryo was stuck. I then had four consecutive miscarriages; the first was a chemical pregnancy (early miscarriage), the second was after a natural conception, and the third and fourth were following IVF. At this point, my husband and I saw PGS as a way of avoiding yet another miscarriage, and FINALLY becoming parents. We decided to move clinic's as our first one, (which we loved), didn't recommend PGS for us, so we commenced with two batching rounds at a clinic where a friend had successfully got a high number of PGS normal embryos. Some clinics recommend PGS testing but many clinics and countries don't, so if it's important to you that your embryos are tested, you need to take this into consideration when choosing a clinic.

After the two batching rounds we discovered all our embryos were abnormal and taking the call for the results was SO hard; much like getting a BFN, (negative pregnancy test), the ground feels like it's opened up beneath you. However, it's a different feeling to getting a negative result after a round of IVF, as there's no transfer – you have the worst of the IVF with the stims, but then the anti-climax of not having the transfer or the hope that you COULD still be pregnant. A double whammy as they say!

We are now going down the egg donation route, and again the question of PGS testing has come up. After our previous experience we've decided it's not for us, and if you do your research from trusted sources, there are as many arguments against testing as there are for it. Ultimately, we went down the PGS route because of my age, as I am in my forties, and the probability of having abnormal embryos increases significantly the older you are. With egg donation, our donor is a lot younger than me and therefore the risks are technically a lot lower.

Wishing you the best of luck whatever route you choose, and sending a million sunbeams and positive vibes for your journey.

* PGS, along with PGD was a term used prior to 2019, nowadays this testing is known as 'Preimplantation Genetic Testing' or PGT, and there are three categories; PGT-A, PGT-M and PGT-SR.

Clare Deakin @iwannabemamabear

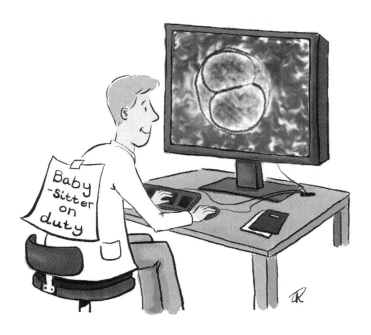

Cartoon of an embryologist viewing a developing embryo

Benefits of IVF affirmations

Includes an excerpt from the blog: 'The power of affirmations'

I always assumed IVF was for women that had 'left it too late,' and egg freezing was for career girls and women that hadn't met 'Mr. Right' in their thirties. I never thought it would take me and my partner of ten years, two and a half years of various fertility treatments - IUI and two fresh IVF cycles - to conceive a baby.

Getting married at twenty-five and trying for a baby at twenty-seven, I thought time was on our side. My husband and I both had a fertility MOT after a year of trying and were told there was nothing that would stop us from falling pregnant naturally. A second-year passed ... still no baby. We made a conscious effort to be healthier, try at the right time of the month. I became ever so slightly obsessed with using OPK's (ovulation predictor kits) religiously each month; we took more 'relaxing' holidays and I started acupuncture and yoga. Still no baby. As the pregnancy announcements came rolling in from friends and friends of friends on social media, I couldn't help but feel completely left behind, helpless. Why was it not happening for us?

Unexplained infertility consumed me. The day we visited a private fertility clinic was the best decision as it felt like we were finally moving forward. After more tests and still no diagnosis, we fell into the 'unexplained infertility' bracket. All I wanted was a logical explanation as to why we couldn't conceive naturally so we could 'fix' it. It took a failed IUI (intrauterine insemination) cycle, and a shambles of an IVF round, resulting in mild OHSS (Ovarian hyperstimulation syndrome) and a chemical pregnancy, to get the answer.

We moved to a new clinic who suggested there was one last test to do; the result confirmed my natural killer (NK) cells were elevated. NK cells are naturally occurring cells which play a vital part in the immune system; the purpose of the cells is to recognize and target other cells which don't belong in the body. Mine were attacking the embryo, leading to implantation failure and miscarriage, (author note: though opinions vary on this).

Finally, with a diagnosis and a new treatment plan, we crossed our fingers that maybe, just maybe, it would work this time. Our second round resulted in seventeen eggs being collected; six made it to blastocyst stage and two were transferred. By comparison, our first round resulted in seven eggs and one blastocyst.

A very long two-week wait later confirmed we were pregnant with Milo. Of course, I was thrilled. But sadly, things didn't get easier from there. With my NK cells still high, I was monitored daily until our six-and-a-half week scan confirmed a heartbeat. I needed a blood test and intralipid drips every three weeks until I was twenty-four weeks pregnant to combat the NK cells, as well as three daily injections until I was twenty-seven weeks pregnant – all to prevent miscarriage.

Finally, on the 2nd July 2019, we welcomed our son into the world by emergency c-section. The best day of our lives. We never gave up hope and would do it all over again for our miracle boy.

Throughout our treatments, my acupuncturist recommended I practice positive affirmations when she picked up on my anxiety after our failed cycles. She gave me a few examples which I repeated aloud five times, once a day.

So, what are positive affirmations? Rather than blanket positive thinking such as: 'today is going to be a good day', affirmations ensure YOU are steering YOUR thoughts, thereby resulting in a hugely beneficial impact, not just on the way you feel but the experiences you have.

IVF can be exciting but the waiting and anticipation can make the process nerve-wracking, causing stress and anxiety. Because of this, it's important to nurture the mind. Benefits of IVF affirmations in particular are:

- Releasing fear

- Letting go of anxiety

- Shifting negative thoughts to positive ones

- Practice being grateful

- Manifesting an outcome

- Attracting good things into your life.

By using positive affirmations as a way of letting go of the negative thoughts weighing you down, you can switch your perspective so you're in control of your thoughts and feelings. Focusing on a positive mind plan can have a positive and powerful outcome on conception. IVF is emotional enough, especially with your body being pumped full of hormones along with the excitement, nerves, and not to mention the two-week wait. I know first-hand how you can transform the experience of feeling like you're on a rickety rollercoaster to feeling strong and powerful. You have the power to change your thoughts as only you know what you're going through.

If you have an upcoming IVF cycle, I've included some examples below. When doing the affirmations, exhale stress and inhale peace:

- **Fear:** The stress is going to make this cycle fail

  Positive affirmation: I am doing everything I can to be my healthiest mentally and physically for this IVF cycle

- **Fear:** I am scared of the impact on my relationship/ marriage

  Positive affirmation: I am in a loving, honest relationship, and my partner/husband loves me no matter what

- **Fear:** I am scared of injections/upcoming procedures

  Positive affirmation: I am strong, focused and

powerful – I can deal with anything

• **Fear:** What if I miscarry?

  Positive affirmation: I put my faith and trust in my body and the power of creation.

You and only you can change your thinking. You have got this mama!

Lisa Penny @fertilityism

(Link to blog: https://www.lisapenny.co.uk/single-post/2019/05/09/The-power-of-positive-affirmations)

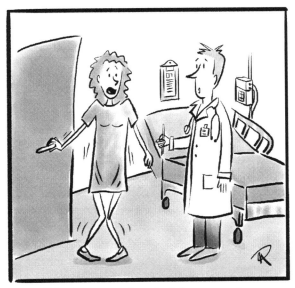

"Now, you absolutely promise
me it won't fall out?"

Things you should know about IVF

Where do I begin? A journey that my husband and I have now been on for over five years. As is common with many couples, we decided that following our marriage we'd take the plunge and start baby-making on our honeymoon. A few months passed and magically we fell pregnant naturally with our first baby. You can only imagine our delight; it was that easy, and even better, a few of our close friends were also pregnant so we could go through it all together. Sadly, for us, this wasn't the reality.

Making a baby isn't as easy as you think. When I was younger it was drummed into you that if you weren't careful, you'd end up pregnant. I wish that was the case. After a year of problems and losses, we approached our GP who referred us for tests. A year later, we were truly blessed to be given the funding for two fresh and two frozen rounds of IVF on the NHS (National Health Service in the UK). Like many others, we went into fertility treatment naively, and thought it would work.

IVF is mind-blowing. It's exhausting and very demanding. Don't be surprised if you don't feel yourself. Some of the medication can impact on your emotional wellbeing. When we did our fresh IVF cycle through scans carried out at our clinic, it was identified that I have polycystic ovaries and would, therefore, respond well to the medication to stimulate my follicles and hopefully produce a good number of eggs. If only I'd known what this would do to me physically: constipation and bloating, leaving me looking six months pregnant by the time egg collection/retrieval day came. My stomach (though the clinic said it was actually my ovaries), felt heavy and painful, and following the collection of thirty-one eggs(!) it really took it out of me. Luckily, I didn't get OHSS (ovarian hyperstimulation syndrome – which can be life-threatening) and managed to recover for our transfer day. Although our embryo attached and we had a positive pregnancy test, we lost our baby shortly after. I then went on to have two frozen embryo transfers which both ended in early miscarriages – and I suffered from palpitations and anxiety – something I'd never experienced before.

The majority of people do IVF whilst working a full-time or part-time job which means fitting in appointments, scans, blood tests, investigations, egg collection (takes a day at least), and embryo transfer, (a day or more depending on how you want to spend your two-week wait), phone calls for results and progress when the eggs have been fertilised. And let's not forget all the research – books, internet, podcasts – to understand all of the above. It's all time-consuming. My bosses were supportive about my appointments, considering it went something like this for our fresh round:

> 1 x consultation appointment to agree our protocol (what would happen and when), and teaching us how to do the injections
>
> 1 x appointment on day 5 for blood tests to see if the drug dosage needed adjusting
>
> 1 x appointment on day 8 for an ultrasound and more blood taken to monitor the growth and number of my follicles
>
> 1 x egg collection - full day off
>
> 1 x embryo transfer - full day off.

Being able to make and receive phone calls during this time, which is weeks rather than a couple of days, is a necessity. My hubby came to the consultation, egg collection and transfer days, so he also had to work this around his job.

I suggest if you are embarking on IVF, think practically and wear comfy clothes that don't constrict your tummy. Also, if like me you bloat, wear something floaty so you don't draw attention to your bump, because the last thing you want is someone suspecting you're pregnant.

We've just been through our seventh pregnancy and are still hoping that one day we'll get to take our little one home. A baby is a miracle that some people create naturally. For others, like my husband and I, it has meant a rollercoaster of emotions and setbacks.

Caren @themissinghare

Take care of your mental health when doing IVF

After three years of trying, testing and dealing with unexplained infertility, the prospect of doing IVF was exciting. I was fit, healthy, happy, in love, and ready to push one out! So down the IVF road we went, figuring it out all on our own. The forms, the testing, the scans, the drugs, the appointments, and of course, the bills.

At the time we were trying to make the most of it, joking and laughing our way to the egg collection room where they retrieved thirteen eggs. But the fun times stopped there. Over the next few days, we found out that six eggs were mature enough to fertilize, but embryo development was poor – so distressing. We transferred two embryos and waited for a miracle. I got my period on Day 28, which was a Sunday when we were in London, away from the comforts of home. I was back to work the next day, and two days later, all the drugs exploded throughout my body.

Emotionally I was a wreck in more ways than one. At this time in my journey, I didn't have any practices in my life that supported my mental health. I got through the hard times by drinking and pretending everything was okay. About a month after our first failed IVF, we found ourselves in London again, sitting under a tree in Hyde Park. A close friend suggested we should change our diet. We were confused. "Really? We're not unhealthy and we don't eat junk food." But we were willing to try anything, so I started to see a health coach.

It turned out that health coaching is so much more than your diet, and that your mental and emotional wellbeing plays an essential part in your overall health. Alongside a Paleo diet, I introduced some mindfulness practices, including yoga and journaling, and used a visualisation meditation app. I found these incredibly hard to do at first, and in all honesty, it took me a very long time to commit to these practices.

Around a year after our failed IVF cycle, we still weren't pregnant, and we still had no answers to our unexplained infertility. We felt a lot healthier, though, so thought we'd give IVF another chance. We left our first clinic and sought out one that was more comforting and used more advanced testing. We felt good about all the changes we'd made in the past year, and it turned out to be a good investment. They collected twelve eggs and five became beautiful looking embryos. We transferred the best-looking one and felt incredibly confident. This time I didn't even make it to Day 28. I was beyond crushed. So much so that I started to look into surrogacy.

The diet and lifestyle changes I'd made before the second failed IVF gave me the strength, and the hope, to keep looking for an answer, to keep fighting for our future family. I took some time to breathe, and at our 'WTF' appointment, we demanded the immune testing we were talked out of when we first went to the clinic. They'd said I wasn't a candidate because I wasn't having recurring miscarriages. And there it was – the answer to my unexplained infertility. My results revealed high NK Cells, (natural killer cells), which meant my body wouldn't let the embryos implant. I put aside the surrogacy papers and with our last scrap of hope, we did our first frozen embryo transfer with the support of immune-suppressing drugs, a clean diet, and my visualisation meditation. Two weeks after the transfer we got the call we'd been waiting on for almost six years. I was pregnant!

Infertility is so demanding on your emotions in every aspect of your life. When you decide to use IVF to help achieve your dreams, it can feel like everything gets amplified by one-hundred. Taking care of your mental health during IVF might be the last thing on your list, but it's the number one thing that's going to get you through the rollercoaster ride you might feel you're on.

Monica Cox @findingfertility

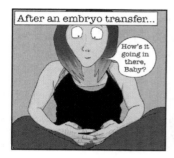 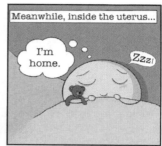

Performance anxiety – 3 days it took!

From an Instagram post

I want to share this with you guys as I've got a lot of new TTC friends this week. My wife's egg collection was on Tuesday, and it wasn't until Friday that I managed to get my sperm sample. Anyone here ever played with a sack of jelly for three days straight? Well, I have! I heard another good saying the other day about this: 'It's like trying to get toothpaste out of an empty tube'.

If this happens to your hubby, don't tell him anything that will put him under further pressure. My wife gave me as much time as I needed, and told me all would be well and that we could freeze sperm and eggs.

You see, it's a knot in the man's brain. They're thinking about something else like eggs, wife in the clinic, bills, cats... who knows. But this block won't disappear until the pressure is off!

Truth is, it was only when I knew my wife was comfortable and having a relaxing bath that the stress was off. I decided to try again and boom! Give your partner space, take the pressure off him, and it will eliminate that mental block in his brain.

We now have our sample and six good eggs ready for our next trip back to Prague.

@the.swim.team (this Instagram account is no longer live, permission was obtained)

IVF feels like you're doing something

After years of trying to conceive (TTC) and after two natural pregnancy losses, we've finally been given the diagnosis of 'unexplained infertility.' We were happy they didn't find anything sinister but at the same time, we wish we knew what was wrong so it can be fixed. And as a result, having sex becomes a chore, which isn't how it should be when you're in your mid to late twenties like me and my husband.

When we finally started IVF (in-vitro fertilisation), I remember thinking: 'This is it, maybe I just need progesterone or oestrogen support, or maybe they just need to pick one good embryo and it will work for us first time'. When I had my first injection at the beginning of the treatment, I felt this overwhelming feeling of comfort as if I was preparing my body for something magical to happen, and getting closer to my dream. All through the soreness from the injections, the mood swings, the hot flushes and all the symptoms the clinic told me about, I kept telling myself I'm doing this for a reason ... to have our baby!

Like most people on their first cycle, I had very little knowledge which, in some ways, I was thankful for as I didn't stress over the results and numbers, such as how thick my womb lining was or how many follicles were growing. But looking back, I wish I knew more about what happens after egg collection as expectations aren't always realised.

Many people think they collect the eggs, put them back into the womb, and job done; it's that easy. Being an IVF baby myself I thought the same, until we went through it ourselves. During egg collection, I remember hearing the embryologist calling out each time an egg was collected from a follicle, which was exciting as we knew we had quite a few. I didn't think of the next step even then. I assumed all the eggs would fertilise as so much emphasis is put on the number of eggs collected.

After egg collection I was transferred to a bed on the ward, and being a healthcare assistant myself, I could hear the embryologist and doctors talking and thought then that something wasn't right. A little later, my husband and I were called into a side room, which terrified me. I knew from previous experiences that this is where they tell you the bad news. The embryologist explained that my husband's sperm wasn't as high a count as it had been previously. They advised to do what's called a 'Split Cycle,' which means half of our embryos would be IVF where the eggs and sperm are left to fertilise with no intervention, and the other half would be fertilised by the embryologist injecting a single sperm into the centre of the egg, otherwise known as ICSI, (Intracytoplasmic Sperm Injection). We were anxious but trusted our embryologist in this decision.

We were lucky enough that seventeen eggs had been collected, but only eight had fertilised, which at the time seemed a huge drop in numbers. I'd been protective over my eggs for the last few months and when they don't survive overnight, it's distressing. They're all your potential babies. Then each day, you wait to hear how many 'embryo babies' are dividing as they don't all carry on developing as they should. Many embryos are transferred back into the womb on day two and successfully become a baby. But many women, myself included, hope they'll develop until day five when they become a blastocyst, because if they aren't transferred, they can be frozen for a future cycle.

I'll never forget waiting for the embryologist to call us each day with an update on our embryos and how they were doing. Even though I was upset that the numbers went down, I always remember someone saying to me: "It only takes one!" And that's still stuck with me.

After regular updates from the embryologist, day five arrived, and we were lucky enough to have six blastocysts – one ready for transfer and five frozen for future embryo transfers.

I'm open about our IVF journey and I've found there's always someone who'll say, "I know someone who had IVF and then got pregnant naturally", or "Congratulations," as if IVF is a given and will work the first time.

Although our next steps are to prep for our fourth transfer, I always tell myself it will be us one day; we will get past the two-week wait; we will get to scan day and hear a heartbeat, and we will hold our baby in our arms. I have really bad days, of course, as it can be a lonely journey. I'm lucky to have a great support system, although, I often feel I don't fit in with my friendship group as some already have children and others don't want a family yet, so they don't understand why I've gone through IVF. It helps me to remember this quote: 'Don't measure your progress with someone else's ruler.'

IVF is an amazing, fascinating journey and it can give you the best chance to have a baby. However, it can also be lonely and difficult, as your emotions fluctuate and you have to stay strong to get through it. The online support I've had has been amazing and I couldn't have got through all my IVF cycles without it.

Although we've been given a diagnosis of unexplained infertility, many people might ask: "So can you still get pregnant naturally?" Yes, of course we can, and every month we wonder whether we are pregnant. In fact, for the past four years I've done a pregnancy test every single month, and the disappointment gets harder, because you build your hopes up and pray that this will be the moment it will happen and we won't have to pursue any more IVF cycles. It breaks my heart when I tell my husband that it's a negative result, and it also takes the fun out of everything because it's all about baby-making. When we did fall pregnant naturally, I knew about five days before my period was due, so every month at the end of my cycle, those five days seem like forever, and every symptom feels like early pregnancy ... but in reality, those feelings are so similar to PMS. And every month, it plays games with our minds.

Katy Jenkins @thejstartshere & ivf_got_this_uk

What your partner needs you to know about dealing with IVF

Based on the blog of the same name.

Fellas, you might think that your contribution to the fertility treatment process ends with providing a sample or two of your little swimmers – but you couldn't be more wrong about IVF. You're not just a bystander. Buckle up buddy, because you and your partner chose to take this crazy ride together. And this is about to get real.

She's going to need you like never before – literally in ways you haven't been prepared for. This is not PMS. This is not a drill. Chocolate and tissues are not going to be enough. In case you weren't already aware, there are going to be good days, bad days, rough patches, good and bad news, and needles – hundreds of fucking needles – taking blood, injecting hormones and, just for fun, you might like to try acupuncture while you throw everything at this menace called 'unexplained infertility'.

So, let's get clear on what she doesn't need from you during IVF (actually ever, but especially now):

- Pity or blame

- Pettiness and frustration

- Pressure in the bedroom

- Pressure to be awesome in every other aspect of her life

- Penny-pinching: because heads up, treatment can quickly get expensive. So, I recommend you set some limits and expectations about the resources you have as a team for your shared goal of parenthood.

What she needs from you:

- Understanding that her body is going to go through the wringer and it's going to drag her mind along for the ride. She's not crazy, she's trying really hard to make you a daddy

- Unity – you're a team in this mess and she needs to feel she is enough for you – with or without a baby. You're already a family

- Unconditional love – a shoulder to cry on, arms to hold her and make her feel safe, loved and supported, even on the darkest days … or for no reason at all

- Unlimited patience for her decisions; empathize with her feelings and discuss with compassion, especially if you experience loss.

And if you do suffer a loss, she'll need unlimited time to grieve, in whatever way she finds healing. Your grief is important too, and your way of grieving will be different to hers, and it's just as necessary for you to grieve your loss, too. So, please, remember to look after yourself whilst you're looking after her. And don't underestimate the power of a good cry, an angry boxing session with a trainer, or writing down your thoughts to clear your head. That goes for both of you.

Ultimately what she really needs is YOU. In her corner. AT ALL TIMES. But especially when:

- Treatments get too invasive, painful or just too much

- Someone makes an insensitive comment about your situation that sets her off

- Your mother asks you again when she's going to be a grandmother

- She knows her body better than anyone – including the doctors – and she needs you to help her stand her ground.

I can't recommend strongly enough that you seek out the support of a professional to help you steer through the choppy waters ahead. It doesn't have to be me, but I'm here for you if you'd like to talk. I see women individually or with their partners, and please believe me when I say the process works much better when couples face things as a team. Fertility is not a "women's problem", it's a family issue and one that's best coped with when supported by our loved ones.

I wouldn't wish fertility struggles on my worst enemy, so don't leave your partner to manage all of this on her own and expect her to present you with a baby at the end of it. It's rough and harsh and you'll both be changed in the process, whether you admit it now or not.

Take care of each other whatever happens.

Much love and baby dust.

Sandi x

Sandi Friedlos @sandifriedlos

(Link to blog: https://sandifriedlos.com/2020/what-partners-need-to-know-about-ivf/)

Yoga helped my sense of well being

Twenty years ago I married a wonderful human being. Our plans were clear: we would work, travel, and then after two to three years, we'd have a baby. We stuck to our plan and then tried to conceive. Suddenly, things didn't go as planned. I wasn't getting pregnant and that's where our journey started. Many tests and treatments, cycle after cycle, feelings starting to bloom … then loss, despair, loneliness, guilt, and unanswered questions: Why me? What's wrong with my body? Is it my fault? Is my partner going to leave if I don't get pregnant? What's my role as a woman if I'm not a mother? The feelings and questions all kept coming …

It was one of the hardest trials of my life: the shots, the hormones, the visits to the doctors, and yet I was blessed to have an amazing husband supporting me and job flexibility to attend all these appointments. At that time in my country (Costa Rica), IVF was prohibited by law, so we did a couple of IUIs (intrauterine insemination) which failed. I discovered I had endometriosis and, as part of the treatment, menopause was induced for six months. I was desperate, twenty-nine years old and menopausal – not a happy experience. Then we did two more IUIs and got pregnant with my lovely boy, who's now sixteen.

We tried for a second child and nothing happened. It was important to me that my son had a sibling to play with, to support each other as they grew older … so my picture of a family wasn't complete yet. 'Secondary infertility' as it's known, can be even lonelier. You're not part of the group of parents without children; you're also not part of a group who feel their families are complete, even with one child. Instead, you feel guilty because you already have a child, yet you're sad.

This time the IUIs didn't work. We did four and I wasn't responding to the medicines. We had to decide if we wanted to do IVF. As previously mentioned, since IVF was restricted in my country, the option was to go elsewhere. This involved decisions at many levels – financial, for example. We'd be gone for at least ten days with a three-year-old, and I had religious beliefs that were causing me concerns.

Eventually, we decided on Colombia and injected the meds whilst still at home. Seven follicles were growing and about four days before the trigger shot for egg retrieval, we left for our adventure. Fortunately, my friend and former business partner lived in Colombia and we were able to stay at her place. The doctors at our clinic were able to extract five ovules (eggs), two of which weren't viable, so we had ICSI (where the sperm is injected into the egg) with the remaining three. Only one fertilized and was transferred. I remembered the doctor said to me: "This is where science ends and it's up to God from this point on. It doesn't matter what you do, if it's meant to be, it will work".

We remained in Columbia for a couple of days. After that my bloodwork showed that my estrogen and progesterone levels were very low, meaning it was likely the ICSI cycle hadn't worked. I began taking high doses of progesterone and estrogen.

Finally, the day came for my pregnancy test and we discovered I was a mum again! Our son was born almost four years after his brother. My family was complete.

During my second pregnancy, I discovered yoga and my sense of wellbeing became a constant in my life, breathing deeply every time anxiety crept in. The acceptance of all the twists and turns became much easier, and the importance of being present in my daily activities was clear as we only have the here and now.

Suddenly, I wanted to share with my loved ones all the gifts the practise of yoga gave me. Eventually, I learned about the mind-body connection and an amazing coaching method to connect with our greatness.

I now understand why I had to go through challenges to have my baby boys. It was a journey to help me connect with couples to ease their fertility struggles. I meet with women weekly, giving them a safe environment to share their feelings and questions. I believe empathy towards these women is one of the greatest gifts given to me.

If you are reading this and feel some connection, remember you're not alone. And I promise things will get better. Take a deep breath every day.

With love,

Carla

Carla @Carlafertility.coach

We've never told anyone we did IVF

My husband and I chose a solitary infertility and IVF journey, but it was the right decision for us. Why? Well, several reasons …

My brother and sister-in-law were already on a waiting list at the same hospital for IVF where we'd been referred. I was confident it would work for us both, but my husband wasn't so sure and recommended we kept our treatment private 'just in case'. Our treatments were literally days apart. So, when we received their picture of a positive pregnancy test only two days after my period came, confirming our unsuccessful cycle, I was relieved they didn't know about us. We were able to genuinely share their joy even though we'd had our own heart-breaking blow.

Besides, my mum hasn't got the best mental or physical health and I didn't feel she'd cope with knowing our challenges as well as my brother's. My dad and his wife came to the end of their IUI and IVF journey, too, and I knew she was struggling with it – so it was best not to tell them either. My husband also felt his family would add pressure to our journey, all out of love and care, but he preferred not to have to deal with their questions.

As we weren't telling family, we decided not to tell friends either. Only a few of my colleagues eventually knew and that was purely because I'd broken down in tears at work. It's funny the conversations you're privy to when people have no idea you're going through IVF. People become 'experts' about fertility treatment, simply because a friend's neighbour's sister went through it. It amused me to hear: "You know, a typical overprotective IVF mum rushes her son off to hospital with just a runny nose". How I chuckled to myself over that one!

Working as a social worker certainly threw a few emotions into the mix. I've accepted that others can and do have children easily, even if they struggle to care for or even abuse them. That's just life. But at times, something would trigger me, leaving me so deeply saddened that I may never experience what they have; life didn't seem to share out luck equally for either me or those abused or neglected children.

There were times I felt I may implode, carrying so much and sharing so little. Close friends faced fertility struggles, too, and I carried a great deal of guilt when they shared their struggles with us, yet said nothing of ours. But in hindsight, I'm glad we kept our journey private. There was no burden of other people's emotions, and I would have hated seeing friends or family eyeball each other or stop conversations so as not to cause upset if talking about pregnancy or babies.

As a Fertility Coach, I appreciate fully the unique choices people make about what they share about their journey. It's not always through shame or guilt, as is often the assumption when people hold back.

We are through the other side of our journey now with two happy and healthy children. Yet, whilst I'm ready to talk about our IVF journey with family and friends, my husband still isn't. I respect and uphold his decision, but for me, I need a full release. He's happy for me to talk to clients or professionals as he sees the benefit of this, but for now, this remains a work in progress.

ANON

Nothing is ever certain when doing IVF

After a couple of years of trying to conceive naturally, my husband and I both had the usual tests to see if there were any problems. The ultrasound scan of my womb came back normal, but there were issues with my husband's sperm test which showed he had no sperm (azoospermia). The only way we'd be able to have a baby was if my husband's sperm was surgically extracted in an operation called 'Micro TESE', which meant we needed to do in-vitro fertilisation or IVF.

With a date in the diary, I wrote a very detailed timing plan and kept busy preparing. I went to see a nutritionist and started exercising and gave up drinking. I wanted to ensure my egg quality was the best it could be. We also spent two agonising months picking a sperm donor, in case his operation failed.

IVF stimulation started and all looked good, although my husband was anxious about his impending operation which would be the day before my egg retrieval. On the morning of his operation, I had to be in a different part of the hospital at 6.30 a.m. for my pre-op, so I said a fleeting goodbye in the taxi. I raced back to his hospital wing but missed seeing him before he went under anaesthetic. I burst into tears. I hadn't had a chance to say goodbye or good luck, knowing how nervous he was. They were the worst few hours of my life.

My father-in-law and I sat in a dingy waiting room whilst time stood still. The surgeon said it would take roughly two hours, but it took five. You can guess the outcome: the surgeon came in with his head hung low and removed his face mask to confirm our worst fears, that the operation hadn't been a success, although they would observe the sperm overnight just in case. My husband was devastated, having been so optimistic and determined. He was also in considerable pain. I was so proud of him and tried to comfort him as much as I could. I was also terrified about the egg collection scheduled for the next morning. We found out ten minutes before I was sedated for my egg collection that my husband's sperm wouldn't be viable, and that the route we needed to pursue was with the donor sperm.

After the egg collection I was in considerable pain, but pleased to have had twelve eggs retrieved. Understandably, that evening we had mixed emotions. The next morning came and it was confirmed that all twelve eggs had fertilised. Wow, I thought, that guarantees a baby, right?

Fast-forward two weeks after the transfer of two, three-day-old embryos, and it's Easter Sunday. The perfect time to test, when you're confident you're pregnant. My husband and I snuck into the bedroom – we were staying with family who had no idea – and despite the nurses saying to wait for the blood test, we tested early that afternoon. We sat nervously watching for the flashing line – until it popped up: 'NOT PREGNANT'. Our worlds came crashing down once again. All that physical and emotional pain, plus expense, and yet, no baby. I panicked thinking were there issues on my side?

Over the next couple of months, I found it hard to socialise and we both felt depressed. The only thing keeping me going was the prospect of trying again with our two frozen blastocyst embryos. I went back to the nutritionist and continued to be as healthy as possible, taking all sorts of fertility-boosting vitamins and powders, which was more expense. This time, I underwent expensive specialist genetic and immunology testing, where they took over twenty syringes of blood. I was black and blue. These tests revealed that I had high natural killer cells and a blood clotting genetic condition called Factor V Leiden. More concern and complications! Despite mixed opinions on whether immunology makes a difference to conception and carrying a baby, the cost to undergo treatment seemed reasonable in comparison to the overall treatment costs; so we went for it.

This was our second attempt with our frozen embryos. I was totally convinced it wasn't going to work and kept saying so to my wonderful specialist who had the nicest bedside manner. "We'll see. No reason why it won't," she said. So, we transferred both frozen embryos.

The two-week wait was such a dark time. I went to see a hypnotherapist to help with my mental state, which truly made me feel more relaxed. Fast forward a few weeks and it was testing time again. My husband banned me from doing a home pregnancy test because the first failed attempt was so awful.

After having my blood test at 7 a.m. that morning feeling terrified and tearful, I had to wait six hours for the results. I answered the phone shaking and immediately blurted out: "It hasn't worked has it?" And the nurse replied: "YES, IT HAS!" I was in total amazement! We then had the pregnancy confirmed by a six-week scan. On 26th February 2017, our first daughter was born. She recently turned two and rocks our world.

Towards the end of my maternity leave, we decided to create more embryos as we didn't have any left. I spent the four months leading up to this fresh cycle of IVF getting back in shape, not drinking, and seeing the same amazing nutritionist to prepare my mind, body and soul. Somehow, this time, I felt even more nervous, maybe because I feared we wouldn't be lucky a second time and I knew how much I wanted to give my daughter a sibling.

In January 2018, the IVF stimulation started all over again. I went nervously into my first consultation, excited about seeing my specialist, who felt like a friend by this point! Instead, I was greeted by a man who didn't have a pleasant bedside manner. He also told me I had fewer follicles than he'd hoped for and to quote him: "Probably because you're older now." I was only thirty-three! I didn't feel I had any luck on my side.

Transfer day came and miraculously three out of eight fertilised embryos were looking great on day 5. Woohoo, transfer time! Again, I assumed this fresh cycle wouldn't work because it hadn't for our very first cycle. Our specialist advised we transfer two embryos because one was doing better than the other. She said the chance of twins was around twenty per cent. We agreed to take her advice. Deep down I was hoping for twins because I knew this could be my last shot at having three children.

Over the next ten days, waiting to test was a complete blur: my hormones were raging and I couldn't stop crying. I couldn't decide whether to wait for the blood test or do an early home pregnancy test. I woke up one morning at 4 a.m. and couldn't get back to sleep. It was three days before I was due in for my blood test. I don't know why but I ran into the bathroom and grabbed the emergency pregnancy test I had lurking in the cupboard, and tested. My heart was pounding, especially as my husband was fast asleep and he'd already told me he didn't want to know if I tested early because of the first home pregnancy test drama.

BANG! Two VERY strong lines appeared immediately, so I did it again with a different pregnancy test, and it came up with 'Pregnant'! I spent the whole weekend buzzing and retesting every few hours. Same result. That following Monday my blood tests confirmed I was pregnant. This time I felt different – my HCG hormone levels came back four times higher than when I was pregnant with our daughter, and I was being physically sick from four and a half weeks as well as waking up in the night starving! There we have it: after nine LONG and extremely hot months during the peak of that summer's heatwave, our twins were born at 37.5 weeks, both healthy and gorgeous. I still pinch myself that it's really happened.

Eloise @fertility_help_hub

Making babies the hard way

The materials to make you
were honed by love
and tried for a long time
even before the investigations,
operations and treatment procedures.

Tried over and over,
like the vials in the carry case
ordered again and again
as fingers shaking for jabs
become steady experts.

The language learned
and abbreviations understood.
At first strange, then familiar,
like the code of life itself,
helix halves becoming whole.

Defrost

I wake early and sit by the phone

for hours, knowing today is the day.

I imagine a stranger holding cloudy vials

of four who will melt transparent into life

or death.

I let it ring four times, a sound for each

- good news and bad.

Two Okay. One looks particularly strong -

growing – the other has lost cells

but it's still alive so worth a try.

I say thank-you and goodbye.

Baby Making Sex

Forum speak…

I am PUPO for now. The

2WW, nightmare-wait for AF to arrive,

yet again, no BMS, AFM so scared of another BFN,

DP says I'm a nightmare at the moment, time is going

so slowly, now 7 DPT – we have a 3-day ET this time,

trying to not look at the HPTs, have six in the cupboard.

Must not test early. This whole TTC thing does

your head in. IF sucks. Am sick of TX.

Afraid of OTD, BFN & M/C

Glossary

2WW = 2 Week Wait (the nail-biting period between embryo transfer/ovulation/basting and pregnancy testing).

AF / Aunt Flo = Menstrual cycle.

AFM = As for me. BFN = Big Fat

Negative. BMS = Baby making sex.

DP = Dear Partner.

DPT = Days past transfer.

ET = Embryo Transfer.

HPT = Home Pregnancy Test.

IF = Infertility.

M/C = Miscarriage.

OTD = Official test day.

PUPO = Pregnant Until Proven Otherwise (i.e. on the 2ww).

TTC = Trying To Conceive.

TX = Treatment.

Justine Bold @justinebold

Making changes as a couple changed our IVF outcome

I was born in Colombia, South America and at the age of thirty-two, I discovered my fallopian tubes were blocked due to severe endometriosis. Even after doing a laparoscopy to try and unblock them, it didn't work, making IVF (in vitro fertilization) the only option. My husband was supportive; however, the emotional stress was heavy on both of us. My first cycle was successful – they retrieved thirty-four eggs and fourteen of them fertilized. I had four embryos transferred and I had a daughter who is now fourteen-years-old.

In 2009, we decided to have a second baby. We weren't worried as our first IVF cycle had been so successful. Secretly, we both desperately wanted a son this time. We started our next cycle, but due to a mistake in the medication dosage made by the clinic, I got OHSS (ovarian hyperstimulation syndrome – where far too many follicles grow and is life-threatening), and my cycle was cancelled. The RE (reproductive endocrinologist) offered us another cycle at no cost.

On my next IVF cycle, we got four embryos, one of which was less developed, but the clinic said we could transfer all four. We made up our minds that the three well-developed embryos were male – they had to be, didn't they? We got a positive pregnancy test and were convinced we were expecting a boy. We decided to find out the sex of the baby at the scan and to our surprise, it was a girl! We hadn't expected that and it took us a few days to accept.

I had a good pregnancy, everything was normal, but no one knew I was developing a blood issue. At thirty-nine weeks, three days before my due date, our baby girl, Isabelle, died in my womb due to a blood clot in the umbilical cord – but I still had to deliver her. Devastated and lost, I felt guilty for what happened, believing it was because I wanted a boy, not a girl. We pursued a fourth round of IVF less than two months later. Again, I got a positive test, but I miscarried at seven weeks. I blamed it on my sadness at the loss of Isabelle, the stress and fear combined with other personal issues.

In 2011, my husband and I felt completely lost and didn't know what our future looked like. Driven by fear and ego, we almost got divorced but chose instead to make some positive changes and stay together.

In 2012, we decided to do our fifth and final round of IVF. This cycle was an amazing experience for us both ... full of love, healthy dialogue and peace which was a direct result of our internal struggles and the shifts we made together as a team. This last round of IVF thankfully resulted in the birth of our second daughter who is now seven-years old.

Monica Bivas @monicabivas

IVF abroad

Wanting another child when I already had two wracked me with guilt. I felt as if I should be satisfied, that I was in some way being ungrateful and selfish, hankering after something I didn't need. I realise now this isn't uncommon, and the fact that we have children doesn't mean we cannot desire more. Those feelings are valid and should be acknowledged without guilt or resentment. I felt the longing so strongly that I went for counselling, feeling there was something 'wrong' with me. I read books and looked online trying to find a way to overcome the emotions turning me upside down. It was affecting my mental health and relationships in many aspects of my life.

Having accepted that this was something I needed to do, and now with the support of my loving and patient husband, we started our journey. Because we already had children we weren't entitled to help from the NHS, so we'd be self-funding, due to needing IVF (in vitro fertilisation) as we'd opted for PGD (pre implantation diagnosis), for personal and health reasons. It was the last chance saloon with age and time not on our side, so better to have tried and failed than never to have had a 'shot.'

As a couple, we're pretty adventurous and this was reflected in our experience which wasn't the 'norm.' However, I'm hoping I may help others to consider alternatives, and give some useful information to aid your decisions.

Knowing we'd have to do IVF abroad, I discovered through research that we needed some initial tests before we could proceed. In the UK, this would cost thousands, so we travelled to Kiev in the Ukraine and our adventure began. We arrived in temperatures of minus 14 and I strolled out of the airport wearing my multi-coloured ski jacket and hat with pom-poms, no doubt looking like Elmer the Elephant. We couldn't read the language at the train station so gave up, opting for a taxi, and once we sat in the outdated vehicle, the non-English speaking driver removed the taxi sign and light.

With almost no verbal communication we sped off down the snow-covered highway. Leaving the city, we soon found ourselves being driven down a dark lane and into a disused funfair. Knowing we had a laptop and quite a bit of cash, my hubby began to think of a 'what if' plan. Then the car stopped and the driver turned around and laughed. He did a U-turn back to the main road, turned right instead of left, and we were finally at our hotel, or rather 'boatel'. A simple mix-up of not knowing your right from your left. I could have kissed the ground. The polite driver helped us with our luggage, shaking our hand with gratitude for our patience. The boatel was a large converted boat on the now frozen river Dnieper where men were fishing, sat on the ice with holes drilled in to drop their lines.

We got a taxi to the clinic, and it was superb, immaculately clean with all the facilities and laboratories for tests to be conducted in one building. It felt welcoming and the staff couldn't have been more helpful. We had our consultant appointment, all the tests and pre-IVF scans, and the results translated into English –

all for a fraction of the price in the UK.

Kiev is close to Chernobyl where they have high levels of infertility and genetic issues, so the consultants have excellent knowledge. However, the city itself along with the climate wasn't the best for a seventeen-day stay, and I learned I'm not a lover of sauerkraut and egg every day for breakfast! This clarified our decision to look elsewhere for IVF treatment.

On returning to the UK, we proceeded to get all our final tests organised, thanks to a helpful team at the local NHS family planning and GUM clinic, along with a GP who did my two-day cycle Luteinising Hormone blood test.

From research and experience, I found that the clinics at the top of the Google search results weren't necessarily the best. I had IVF treatment over five years ago and since then communication has got easier and treatment more accessible. Many of the barriers, from translating prescriptions to international delivery of medicines are much easier now, and there's more choice. And along with virtual face-to-face consultations and clinic tours, you don't have to travel to make a decision unless you want to.

The small clinic I eventually chose was in Northern Cyprus which enabled me to build up a good rapport with the consultant. He was open to suggestions of how I wanted to plan my cycle, accommodating mine and my partner's wishes as fully as possible.

If you're considering travelling abroad to do fertility treatment, here are some considerations to think about before you decide on your clinic:

- Check the exchange rate for value when negotiating prices with the clinic. Some parts of your fertility treatment in the UK or your own country, which are added extras, may be included at no extra cost. Ensure your travel insurance covers you adequately for fertility treatment and check your clinic's insurance too.

- You can have all your monitoring done at a clinic that's local to where you live before you go abroad for treatment

- Whist on the stimulating drugs, you need to stay out of the sun which isn't easy in a sunny climate, and you mustn't use the swimming pool. You'll need a sharps box for all the needles and a small one for travelling. Remember to carry your medical details and paperwork to explain to customs if needed. If carrying cash, again have justification, as on return from Cyprus when we didn't complete the cycle, we had to state at the airport why we were carrying so much money.

- If you stimulate before flying, don't do the trigger shot until you arrive in the country where the clinic is. This is crucial because if your plane is delayed, you risk a wasted cycle. When we arrived in Cyprus in the early hours of the morning, we had a team of nurses waiting at the clinic with a warm welcome and my trigger injection.

- It goes without saying, whether your clinic is in your home country or abroad, that you trust and have a good relationship with them. For us, it was important to have twenty-four-hour access to the clinic. The consultants and nurses were contactable by telephone or video call 24/7. The clinic was amazing: clean and professional with all aspects of treatment carried out on the one site. There were beautiful treatment rooms and an English-speaking doctor and nurse, which helped us feel fully informed, safe and comfortable.

On my first cycle, I didn't respond well and was advised in Cyprus to abandon it. It was disappointing but I valued the doctor's professional judgement. I felt sad that I'd put in so much effort and it hurt physically and emotionally, but where there's possibility, there's also hope. I wasn't deterred. At each stage of the journey, I was learning and feeling more prepared. However, I would have been grateful for more information from someone who'd experienced something similar already. The upside of the cycle being cancelled meant I could finally enjoy the waterpark with the rest of the family.

The next cycle resulted in a negative pregnancy test after the dreaded two-week wait, but the following cycle was a positive pregnancy result and because we'd done PGD, we knew we were having a girl. On the second test to check my hormone levels, we found out they hadn't risen as they should, and although I continued with the medication to try and sustain the pregnancy, nature had other plans and sadly I miscarried. Hard as that is to accept, it's often for a reason.

I grieved for the loss, the failure, and the feeling of emptiness. I only had my memories and photos of the embryos and scans; science having made these treasures possible. The embryos were cared for so gently and watched over for many hours in anticipation; the love for something so tiny with so much hope bestowed upon them.

Some six years after this journey began, we were blessed with a natural, healthy pregnancy, despite sickness from the start. I just knew this was it! As I was now a few years older, we opted for a NIPT test in early pregnancy. This was a blood test carried out in the first trimester to discover if the baby had any genetic related health abnormalities. Back then the test was sent to China, but it's now more readily available in the UK, and I would hope may soon be available as a matter of course to all mothers as part of their twelve-week prenatal care. Doing this simple test meant I could avoid having an amniocentesis much later in pregnancy which brings its own risks to the mother and baby, plus the emotional rollercoaster of worry that comes with it.

Eventually, at just over twelve weeks pregnant, I knew I was carrying a healthy baby girl without any genetic risk factors. A pink one, for the first time! I was speechless! She completed our brood and with some science, mother nature, patience, and love, she was born on 12th December 2014, weighing in at a robust 7lb 12.5oz. She rocked our world and still does.

Fertility journeys are not merely a physical struggle but are also hugely emotional. More attention should be given to the impact on your mental and emotional health and a holistic mind/body approach should be considered. My knowledge has continued to accumulate as I studied to become a specialist fertility coach and now help couples with their dreams of becoming parents.

Jo Sinclair @jo.sinclair.resilience.reborn

Four years and four IUIs ended with divorce

The first month of trying to conceive, I experienced nausea and an increased sense of smell right after ovulation. I thought I must be pregnant. After the two-week wait, when the pregnancy test was negative, I was quite confused. And then my period started the next day. On my next cycle I had the same symptoms but again my period arrived on time. I started to think there was something wrong but people told me not to worry and to just keep trying.

However, after a couple more cycles of the same thing happening and no-one believing me, I decided to see some specialists. I saw a naturopath, acupuncturist, and doctor; each time sharing my story and being told that I wouldn't have any symptoms until implantation. I was told it was all in my head because I "wanted to be pregnant so bad".

As more time passed, I started to develop a fear of having pregnancy symptoms and I started to question my intuition. It led me to suffer in silence, instead seeking answers online such as the supportive community through the Resolve message boards. To distract myself from talking about babies and children, I started to take dance classes and go to evening events.

Two and a half years went by and I still hadn't seen a positive pregnancy test, so we went to a fertility clinic. After tests showed mild sperm issues, we did our first IUI (intrauterine insemination). Again I had the same symptoms of increased sense of smell and nausea, but my period arrived on time. While looking for answers, I came across the book *The Infertility Cure* by Randine Lewis, where I read about implantation failure and was surprised to read that other symptoms I was also experiencing - night sweats, early morning insomnia and panic attacks around the time of my period - was my body fighting off an embryo implanting. I had assumed these feelings were due to the emotional rollercoaster of infertility. I wondered what was causing my autoimmune system to be on hyper-alert?

Four months later, we did our second IUI cycle. During the two-week wait I had the same symptoms and this time I told my husband, but he said he couldn't get his hopes up again until we got a positive pregnancy test. This time however, sixteen days after the IUI my period hadn't arrived.

I had blood drawn for my HCG (human chorionic gonadotrophin hormone or pregnancy hormone) levels the next day and waited for the result from the clinic. The phone rang.

"It doesn't look good."

I was confused. "Am I pregnant or not?"

"Technically 'yes' you are pregnant, but your HCG should be higher by now."

Next came two weeks of blood tests to check that my HCG levels were rising; they were, which would indicate the pregnancy was progressing. I gave blood for the seventh test, and sometime later I went to the toilet and noticed that I had started to bleed. Concerned, I called the clinic and they checked through previous results which showed my levels had been doubling as expected, but the last result, the levels hadn't increased as much. This wasn't a good sign. They said they'd call me the next day with the results of today's blood draw.

Upset at this news I called my husband who was still at work.

He didn't seem concerned and went on to say he'd be staying at his dad's house instead of coming home. Trying to hold back the tears, I suggested he see his dad the next day but he wouldn't and said I should go hang out with a friend.

The next day the clinic said I needed to have an early scan, and this time I was super direct and told my husband he had to take the day off work and come with me to the appointment. He did. While waiting for the scan the bleeding increased and I was doubled over in pain. My husband put his arm around me and looked quite worried but didn't say much. After a short time, a nurse walked through the waiting room, took one look at me and led me to a vacant room. I gave another blood sample and shortly after we had the ultrasound scan.

"We can't find anything in your uterus. I'm sorry but there's no baby."

"Is the baby in my tube?"

"We don't know where the baby implanted, but based on your blood draw we just did, your HCG is still rising. We can't let you miscarry on your own even though you have started bleeding because it could put your life in danger."

After this they gave me a shot of methotrexate. The fertility clinic explained that we wouldn't be able to have any fertility treatment for three months as the drug takes that long to work its way out of my system. But no one talked about the grief surrounding miscarriage or how to deal with the loss as a couple. I rested for a few days; the methotrexate made me feel sick, I was bleeding, depressed and constantly in tears.

We did two more IUIs which brought more disappointment and we realized our marriage needed work. The marriage counselor we saw suggested we each deal with our grief in separate sessions.

Neither one of us felt a connection to her, so looked for someone else. Several people I knew recommended a coach, and although this wouldn't be covered on our insurance, he specialized in anxiety issues and as my husband had previously been diagnosed with clinical anxiety, it made sense to see him. I also hoped he might be able to help me with the emotional trauma I had from trying to conceive.

He used hypnotherapy and visualization which helped me to celebrate my pregnancy whilst also mourning the loss of my baby. He started to work with me to unravel my feelings of inadequacy and failure that surrounded infertility. Through the work I did with him I also looked at other areas of my health that I thought could be affecting my fertility.

There were several things that the coaching helped me with:

1. Knowing that I wasn't alone and to remember that my intuition should be trusted.

2. Allowing for grief enabled me to restore the connection to my intuition.

3. Connecting me to a network of holistic providers helped me to uncover some toxicity in my dental work, and

4. I learned to stop taking responsibility for my husband's emotions and give his energy back to him, so that I'd be free to take care of myself.

Through working with a naturopath, acupuncturist, cranial-sacral therapist, a holistic dentist and taking a long list of supplements, my health started to improve – I was sleeping better and I started to think clearly again. My auto-immune problems began to ease as my body got rid of the toxins.

I had been seeing the coach for six months yet my husband still hadn't attended his first appointment, making excuses each time I asked. Finally, when he came home from his first session, he looked like a weight had been lifted from his shoulders. He said, "I realize that if I were single, I wouldn't want a child. But I'm with you, so let's just go ahead."

As our infertility dragged on, I felt that he didn't really want to be a father because of the way he acted and his comments. But because I so clearly desired with all my heart to be a mother, he didn't want to admit this. He went to some acupuncture sessions but resisted trying other suggested approaches and supplements.

Going through infertility and loss can have a negative effect on a couple's relationship or it can bring a couple closer together. According to a Danish study*, couples who went through fertility treatments that weren't successful were three times as likely to get a divorce. We ended up being one of those couples.

After four years of struggling to get pregnant and stay pregnant, I felt a new sense of loss. I felt healthier than I ever had and thought my body would be more fertile, but I was single. I met my now-husband while swing dancing soon after my divorce, but we didn't date until four years later. Five months after I moved to Sweden to be with him, we conceived naturally when I was forty-three and he was thirty-seven. Our rainbow baby was born in 2016.

*https://www.usnews.com/news/articles/2014/01/31/study-infertile-couples-3-times-more-likely-to-divorce

Leah Irby @leahirby

RESOURCES

Aysha O'Connor is a Health Coach with the Institute of Integrative Nutrition and a Freedom Fertility Formula Specialist. Having been through her own infertility struggles, she's passionate about supporting and guiding women through the emotional pain of infertility. Having used "food as medicine" to conceive her children naturally over the age of 40, she now helps women to improve their reproductive health and boost their fertility, in order to conceive naturally. She specializes in women who are over 35 years of age and dealing with "unexplained infertility."

If you would like to connect with Aysha:

Website www.fertilitywithaysha.com

Becky Kearns is mum to three donor egg conceived daughters and is very open about her infertility story – early menopause, numerous IVF cycles and loss – in the hope that she can inspire and support others who need to consider donor eggs to have their family. She blogs about infertility and having donor conceived children and her hope is that by speaking openly, both IVF and donor conception within society will become much more open and an accepted way of starting a family.

If you would like to connect with Becky:

Instagram @definingmum

Website www.definingmum.com

Caren is a mum to Alessio, who was born too early at 21 weeks and 6 days, and mum to her six other children, all born too soon. She raises awareness of baby loss and infertility as a blogger.

If you would like to connect with Caren:

Instagram @themissinghare

Carla Heilbron is a Human Development Coach from the MMK Institute, Miami, USA, where she currently teaches. She is also a Yoga Teacher and has qualifications in Yoga for Fertility Level I and II in the USA and Canada. For several years she has worked with hundreds of women, sharing the benefits of yoga, breathing and being present. She focussed on working with women dealing with infertility, by helping them find a balance and connection through the mind, body and spirit, to feel empowered and at peace. She has worked with clients in various countries using online tools, and is fluent in English and Spanish.

If you would like to connect with Carla:

Instagram @carlafertility.coach

Website www.carlafertilitycoach.com

Facebook carlafertilitycoach

Chiemi Rajamahendran is an infertility trauma and loss coach offering individual, couples and group support sessions via teletherapy worldwide. Her counselling is tailored to those experiencing stress and anxiety related to infertility, loss and related procedures, such as IVF/IUI. Her support sessions offer a safe, self-reflective, non-judgmental space, no matter what stage of your journey you might find yourself in.

If you would like to connect with Chiemi:

Instagram @missconceptioncoach

Website www.missconceptioncoach.com

Claire Ingle is an advocate for positive culture and wellbeing in the workplace. She wants to use her wide experience in the field of HR and her personal interest in mental health, to influence and change the landscape of how infertility is recognised and responded to by employers.

If you would like to connect with Claire:

Instagram @ivfatwork and @fertilitymattersatwork

Website www.fertilitymattersatwork.com

Dany Griffiths is the founder and creator of the Freedom Fertility Formula. She has been supporting couples with fertility issues since 2007, and has provided mentoring for specialists working in the area of fertility, pregnancy and birth since 2013. She believes the impact of infertility goes way beyond the struggle to get pregnant and have a longed-for baby, yet the importance of supporting mental health and emotional wellbeing is often overlooked. Sadly, this emotional devastation also has the potential to affect the chances of those struggling from becoming pregnant to. Dany is on a mission to change this.

If you would like to connect with Dany:

Instagram @freedomfertilityformula

Website www.DanyGriffiths.com

Email dany@freedomfertilityformula.com

Devon Baeza is The Fertility Finance Coach. She combines her degrees in Finance, Investments, and Master Life Coach training with her years of fertility treatment to help women make savings and manifest money. A self-proclaimed 'money mindset nerd' and lover of spending psychology, her mission is to make sure money doesn't stop anyone from motherhood. She believes that the challenges infertility presents are the perfect time to deal with money blocks once and for all, to not only help women create their future families fast, but to change their financial legacy for life.

If you would like to connect with Devon:

Instagram @the_fertility_finance_coach

Facebook @TheFertilityFinanceCoach

Email Devon@DevonBaeza.com

Website www.devonbaeza.com

Eloise, who experienced a difficult road to motherhood first-hand, decided to set up 'Fertility Help Hub', the fertility lifestyle hub and directory; 'an oasis of fertility'. Sign up to the newsletter for tips, support guidance and inspiration. She wants to help break the stigma around infertility, so people don't have to suffer in silence and spend hours on Google, feeling overwhelmed.

If you want to connect with Eloise:

Instagram @fertility_help_hub,

Facebook fertilityhelphub

Website www.fertilityhelphub.com

Erin Bulcao is 35 years old and originally from Mexico City but now lives in Encinitas CA. She has twin eight-and-a-half-year-old girls conceived through IUI, who are her world but who also test her daily. She's a certified yoga teacher and was teaching at Core Power Yoga but has taken a break whilst going through IVF for the last two-and-a-half years. She's obsessed with NYC and travels there a few times a year because she loves it so much. She met her husband when she was twenty-two, outside of a bar and has been married for ten years! She recently started a blog which has helped her tremendously, and hopes it's also helped others either going through infertility and those wanting to learn more. She's a 'snacker', could eat dessert all day, is a Bravo TV junkie and always has a bowl of cereal before bed.

If you would like to connect with Erin:

Instagram @mybeautifulblunder

Blog www.mybeautifulblunder.com

Jessica Hepburn is one of the UK's leading patient voices on fertility, infertility, the science of making babies and modern families. Having been through eleven rounds of IVF, she understands what it's like to struggle to create the family you long for. She is the founder of Fertility Fest, (www.fertilityfest.com) the arts festival dedicated to fertility, as well as the author of The Pursuit of Motherhood and 21 Miles. She has also swum the English Channel, run the London Marathon and is currently training to climb Mount Everest, all to raise awareness of the mental and physical struggle of infertility and IVF.

If you would like to connect with Jessica:

Instagram @jessica_hepburn_

Website www.jessicahepburn.com

Facebook jessicahepburnauthor

Twitter @jessicapursuit

Jo Sinclair is a Freedom Fertility Formula Specialist and supports women and couples through counselling, coaching and mind/body techniques, to regain emotional control of their fertility journey and enhance their chances of fertility success.

If you would like to connect with Jo:

Instagram @jo.sinclair.resilience.reborn

Website www.resiliencereborn.com

Julianne Boutaleb of Parenthood in Mind is a specialist psychologist and has her own practice for parents and parents-to-be, wherever they are in their journey to parenthood.

If you would like to connect with Julianne:

Instagram @parenthoodinmind

Website www.parenthoodinmind.co.uk

Justine Bold has personal experience of infertility as she had a twelve year journey to motherhood, finally becoming a mum to twin boys in her forties. She has written articles on infertility and edited a book entitled: Integrated Approaches to Infertility, IVF and Recurrent Miscarriage that was published in 2016. She's also co-written a book on mental health that was published in 2019. She works as a University Lecturer and has research interests in lifestyle and nutrition and their links to health problems, such as endometriosis and polycystic ovarian syndrome.

If you would like to connect with Justine:

Twitter @justineboldfood

Instagram @justinebold

Website https://www.worcester.ac.uk/about/profiles/justine-bold

Katy Jenkins is twenty-eight years old and is married to Thomas, who's thirty. They live in Exeter, Devon in the UK with their fur-baby Stan. They have been TTC for five years and have experienced natural losses and failed IVF transfers. They have found social media TTC accounts extremely helpful and supportive during their journey. They decided to create a fertility sock company called 'The Journey Starts Here' with the hope that their socks will bring joy to such an incredibly hard journey. They also think it's a great way to tell your story via social media and to connect with other men and women who understand the struggles of infertility. Katy also treats them as her lucky socks too.

If you would like to connect with Katy and Tom:

Instagram @thejstartshere

Website www.thejourneystartshere.co.uk

Kelly and her husband were an 'older couple' when they had their first ICSI cycle due to male factor infertility. Now the mother to their daughter, she blogs about infertility and motherhood after IVF.

If you would like to connect with Kelly:

Instagram @ivf.ninja

Blog www.motherhoodafterivf.com

Email ivf.ninja@gmail.com

Leah Irby is the creator of Courageous Pregnancy: practices to calm the mind and strengthen the body. She also writes custom songs for pre-conception, pregnancy and loss. She's a certified fertility coach and a music educator who has lived in the US, India, and Sweden. She had an ectopic pregnancy at six weeks and was told at thirty-seven that she wouldn't conceive without IVF. She conceived her son naturally and gave birth to him when she was forty-three.

If you would like to connect with Leah:

Instagram @leahirby

Facebook @newconceptionsbyleahirby

Online courses https://bit.ly/naturalanxietyrelief

SoundCloud @leahirby

YouTube http://bit.ly/leah-irby-YouTube

Lisa Penny and her husband struggled with infertility for two-and-a-half years, undertaking numerous fertility treatments including clomid, IUI and two fresh IVF cycles, before conceiving in October 2018. They welcomed their son into their life on 2nd July 2019. Lisa's fertility journey and passion for health and nutrition inspired her to qualify as a nutrition coach in 2018. She specialises in pre-conception nutrition, sharing her knowledge with clients to conceive naturally and/or alongside assisted fertility treatment.

If you would like to connect with Lisa:

Instagram @fertilityism

Website www.lisapenny.co.uk

Lisa White, OTR/L is an IVF Mentor providing personalized coaching support to those in search of guidance as they navigate the emotional rollercoaster of IVF. Her first book, *Hold On, Baby! - A Soulful Guide to Riding the Ups and Downs of Infertility and IVF* was published in June 2020. She is active on Instagram.

If you would like to connect with Lisa:

Instagram @IVF.manifesting.a.miracle

Website www.ivfmanifestingamiracle.com

Facebook IVF Manifesting A Miracle.

LinkedIn Lisa White

Monica Bivas went through multiple IVF treatments – including the stillbirth of her second daughter – but was determined to try one last time. This time, however, she decided to approach her treatment with mindfulness and positivity which resulted in the birth of her third daughter. She now helps her tribe consciously direct their IVF experience by managing their emotions, shifting their mindsets, and preparing for the ultimate outcome of treatment – a precious baby. She is a regular contributor to the Huffington Post, and has published *The IVF Planner*, a journal and guide for women undergoing fertility treatment, and has another book forthcoming about her life-changing experience with IVF treatment. She is married to her amazing Israeli husband, Shai, whom she considers her best friend, and has two daughters and one step-daughter. Although born in Colombia, she is deeply in love with her home in Long Island, New York. When not supporting her IVF tribe, she fully immerses herself in being a hands-on mom, and a must in her life is a weekly date with her husband doing one of her favorite activities: dancing.

If you would like to connect with Monica:

Instagram @monicabivas

Facebook monicabivasIVFcoach

Facebook Group Theivfjourney

Twitter @MonicaBivas

Pinterest @monicabivas

Website www.monicabivas.com

LinkedIn monicabivas

Monica Cox FDN-P is somewhat of a hippy and is a bit obsessed with real food. Her clean eating lifestyle evolved slowly during her nine-year infertility journey. She spent six years searching for an answer to her unexplained infertility, which included never seeing a BFP and two failed IVFs. She decided to make some dramatic diet and lifestyle changes to improve her fertility health and requested immune tests, even though the doctors told her she wasn't a candidate for such testing. The results came back and she discovered she had high natural killer cells - she believes this was the answer to her unexplained infertility. With five embryos on ice she did three

FETs (frozen embryo transfers), with immune supressing drugs, which resulted in two miscarriages and one beautiful baby boy. Two months after all medical treatment was done and dusted, she found out the dramatic diet and lifestyle changes had paid off and she was pregnant naturally, for the first time ever. Baby boy number two entered their family in March 2018. Monica is a stay at home mom, wife, Fertility Health Coach, author of *Baby & Me*, Podcast host of Finding Fertility and creator of #gratedvegbrekkie. She's all about inspiring others to improve their physical and mental health.

If you would like to connect with Monica:

Instagram @findingfertility

Website www.findingfertility.co

Natalie Silverman had her own fertility journey and is the founder and host of the brilliant Fertility Podcast, where she aims to empower women and men trying to start or complete their families with expert interviews and real-life stories. She is also co-founder of @fertiltymattersatwork with Claire (@ivfatwork) and Becky (@definingmum) and is a Freedom Fertility Specialist, supporting people with their emotional wellbeing.

If you would like to connect with Natalie:

Instagram and Twitter @fertilitypoddy

Website www.thefertilitypodcast.com

Rachael Casella is Mum to her three shooting stars; Mackenzie, Bella and Leo. Mackenzie was diagnosed when she was ten weeks old with a terminal genetic illness called spinal muscular atrophy (SMA) type 1. She only had months to live. Rachael later had a termination of a subsequent pregnancy due to a genetic defect and has done IVF with PGD and PGS to have a healthy sibling for Mackenzie. She is a blogger and genetic carrier testing campaigner, responsible for a historic change in Australia's genetic testing laws. She is the author of *Mackenzie's Mission* – a story of her daughters, her struggles with conception, pregnancy, genetic defects and ultimately death.

If you would like to connect with Rachael:

Instagram @mylifeof_love

Website www.mackenziesmission.org.au

Rachel Cathan is the author of the book: *336 Hours* – a diary of one woman's battle through infertility and IVF during her five-year quest for motherhood. The story is set within the pressure cooker of the narrator's third, and supposedly final, IVF treatment. Rachel is also a fertility counsellor.

If you would like to connect with Rachel:

Instagram @rachelcathancounselling

Website www.rachelcathancounselling.com

Sandi Friedlos supports women and their partners through the emotional and mental strain of fertility struggles and infertility treatment, so they are free from feeling their life is 'on hold' while playing the waiting game. Having survived it too, Sandi knows this stuff is hard and painful, and the people going through it need compassion and a safe space to deal with it all honestly. Sandi hates seeing people suffer and feels drawn to help where she can. But she doesn't believe that holding pretty rocks or thinking positively is enough to help someone get, (or stay) pregnant. She focuses instead on the practical, easy and nurturing things that her clients can do to improve their chances of a successful pregnancy, without sacrificing their relationships and careers in the process. When she's not working, Sandi can be found actively avoiding housework, in her garden harvesting fresh veggies, singing badly in traffic between her kids' over-scheduled extracurriculars or bingeing on Netflix comedy specials with Dave, her lifetime partner in crime.

If you want to connect with Sandi:

Instagram @SandiFriedlos

Website www.sandifriedlos.com

Email sandi@sandifriedlos.com

Facebook SandiFriedlos

Twitter @SandiFriedlos

Sophie Martin is a Registered Midwife and infertility and baby loss advocate. Currently navigating the bumpy road of IVF, whilst also honouring the memory of her twin sons Cecil & Wilfred, after their very premature birth and death. She is dedicated to celebrating the power of women, and acknowledging how important it is to support other women on their journeys to motherhood.

If you would like to connect with Sophie:

Instagram @the.infertile.midwife

Blog www.theinfertilemidwife.com

Suzanne Minnis experienced three failed IVF cycles that left her devastated and wondering if she would ever become a mum. On their fourth cycle, Suzanne and her husband got their BFP, and she is now mama to their miracle daughter. She now blogs about fertility, IVF and motherhood.

If you would like to connect with Suzanne:

Instagram @the_baby_gaim

Blog www.thebabygaim.com

Thank you for buying this book

It means a lot to me and the contributors that we are helping and supporting you.

Please would you do one thing to help people in the same community as you? If you found this book helpful, would you spread the word by leaving an honest review on the website that you brought it from, as this helps others to find the book and provides social proof. Alternatively, you can leave a review on my website here: www.mfsbooks.com Please also feel free to review the book on your own social media channels.

I love to hear from readers and receive feedback about the This is series, after all the books are for people on the same journey as you, so please contact me at sheila@mfsbooks.com

I'm very passionate that people who haven't experienced fertility treatments understand how it really is, because then they will be in a better position to offer the best kind of support. If you agree, why don't you gift a copy to a family member or friend, especially if you want them to know what you're going through but can't bring yourself to tell them personally.

If you are a professional working in a fertility clinic or in your own practice and would like to gift the paperback or ebook to your clients, please contact me at the above email address for discount information.

If you have a podcast or need guest posts for your website, I am always happy to share my story so that it may help others. Just drop me an email.

Don't forget to check out all the other books in the This is series, and my standalone book My Fertility Book, all the fertility and infertility explanations you will ever need, from A to Z – please see my website www.mfsbooks.com for more details.

Don't forget, I make a small donation from this sale to an

appropriate charity in your country. This is the case for all my books.

Wishing you all the very best on your journey to meet your baby.

Love Sheila x

Made in the USA
Las Vegas, NV
03 November 2020